A New Holistic-Evoluti
to Pediatric Palliative C

Carlo V. Bellieni

A New Holistic-Evolutive Approach to Pediatric Palliative Care

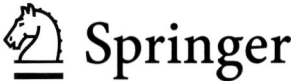

Carlo V. Bellieni
Pediatric Pain Prevention Unit
University of Siena
Siena, Italy

ISBN 978-3-030-96258-6   ISBN 978-3-030-96256-2 (eBook)
https://doi.org/10.1007/978-3-030-96256-2

© The Editor(s) (if applicable) and The Author(s), under exclusive license to Springer Nature Switzerland AG 2022
This work is subject to copyright. All rights are solely and exclusively licensed by the Publisher, whether the whole or part of the material is concerned, specifically the rights of translation, reprinting, reuse of illustrations, recitation, broadcasting, reproduction on microfilms or in any other physical way, and transmission or information storage and retrieval, electronic adaptation, computer software, or by similar or dissimilar methodology now known or hereafter developed.
The use of general descriptive names, registered names, trademarks, service marks, etc. in this publication does not imply, even in the absence of a specific statement, that such names are exempt from the relevant protective laws and regulations and therefore free for general use.
The publisher, the authors and the editors are safe to assume that the advice and information in this book are believed to be true and accurate at the date of publication. Neither the publisher nor the authors or the editors give a warranty, expressed or implied, with respect to the material contained herein or for any errors or omissions that may have been made. The publisher remains neutral with regard to jurisdictional claims in published maps and institutional affiliations.

This Springer imprint is published by the registered company Springer Nature Switzerland AG
The registered company address is: Gewerbestrasse 11, 6330 Cham, Switzerland

Preface

What does pediatric palliative care need to live up to the arduous task they have? We can call it with the expression "being synoptic" (from the Greek words "syn" that means "together" and "ops" that means "to see"), that is, the ability of looking over the whole situation, and at the same time, that of looking together with the patient. A synoptic medicine is able to watch the whole and to watch together.

Synopsis 1: Looking over the whole situation. You will learn not to see just the detail, but the whole picture, and the strategy to follow becomes simpler. Therefore, this text refers to a holistic method of treatment, that is, something that does not say only how to deal with drug therapy or interview techniques, and above all it's not a manual on how to do it.
Synopsis 2: To look together with the patients. You will learn to peer them, putting yourself at the level where you and them can communicate. Communication is not a matter of "how" or "what," but a matter of watching and acquaintance.

Too often we are overwhelmed by lessons on how to approach patients in difficult sets: approach techniques and all the consequent strategies and tricks. But the medical art is not a series of methods and techniques: otherwise, what we do overshadows how we do it. It is the defeat of medicine if we feel okay when we have respected the points prescribed by the protocol or the manual on communication. We expect more from pediatric palliative care. Above all, we expect a common journey with people who are experiencing this hard moment of their lives.

In this book, we will learn this "being synoptic": watching together the various approaches to the disease as a whole and watching together with compassion the patient and their family. This is the aim: learning the sense of the word "together."

We will deal with drugs and treatments, but with the aim of introducing them into a broader sight that does not limit healing to procedures and protocols. And of experiencing how we can do this together with the patients, exploring their mental development, their mood, and preferences. We will also explore the secrets of those parts of bioethics, philosophy, and psychology that are the fundaments of a good medical treatment: here they are not an appendix of a book, as it happens elsewhere, but a pillar of the vision this book stands for.

We will learn how to guarantee children's health even when in the fury of the disease and even in the dark room of depression, because health is not just the absence of a disease. We will also learn how to treat pain; pain does not have only the response to the symptom as its commitment. In short, a synoptic gaze, which is neither the myopic gaze of those who see only a detail, nor the presbyopic gaze of those who look from afar with detachment and sometimes a pinch of cynicism to save themselves from the pain they see.

This is why the title of this book includes the terms "holistic" and "developmental": holistic indicates the whole person and the whole situation; developmental indicates the need of being companions to the patients and of following their needs and requests according to their developmental stage. And when we say "developmental," we do not indicate only the age, but also their process and development of illness, mood, and of bereavement. We want to learn to watch like this, to accompany people like this, and to look at ourselves like this.

Siena, Italy   Carlo V. Bellieni

Contents

Part I Pediatric Palliative Care: "Fundamentalia"

1 The First Obstacle Is in the Handle 3
  1.1 Team-Hierarchy Responsibilities 3
  1.2 Are Doctors Unhappy? 3
  1.3 The Conundrum of Motivation 4
  References 6

2 Palliative Care Is Not a Synonym of End-of-Life Care 7
  2.1 What Is Palliative Care? 7
  2.2 Cultural Resistances 8
  2.3 Heterogeneity of Pediatric Cases 8
  2.4 The Prophecy of Florence Nightingale 9
  References 11

3 Neonatal and Perinatal Care 13
  3.1 Three Paradoxes 13
    3.1.1 First Paradox: Little Bodies Do Not Mean Little Grief ... 13
    3.1.2 Second Paradox: Little Bodies Do Not Mean Little Pain ... 14
    3.1.3 Third Paradox: Small Age Does Not Mean Small Rights ... 15
  3.2 Perinatal Palliative Care 16
  References 17

Part II Communication with Children and Their Families

4 Words Can Break My Heart 23
  4.1 Crucial Importance of the Interview 23
  4.2 The False Myth of Empathy 24
  4.3 Certain News Is Indelible 25
    4.3.1 Silence 26
    4.3.2 The Informed Consent 26
  References 27

5 Managing Grief and Its Phases 29
  5.1 The Phases of Grief 29
  5.2 The Pathological Grief 29

vii

		5.3 Communicating with the Depressed Child or Parent.	32
		5.4 The Experience of Loss	32
		5.5 The Risk of Suicide	34
		5.6 Interventions Aimed at the Family.	34
		5.7 Interventions Aimed at Caregivers.	34
		References.	35
6	**Challenges in Communication with Parents and Children.**	37
	6.1	It Is Difficult to Use the Word Death.	37
	6.2	… Much More That of a Child	38
	6.3	Should We Talk of Their Death and Disease?	39
	6.4	Speaking According to the Patient's Character	40
	6.5	Obstacles to Communication.	41
	6.6	What Helps in Communicating Bad News on Their Health to the Children?.	43
	6.7	Special Children.	44
		References.	45
7	**The Models of Mental Growth.**	49
	7.1	Changes of Comprehension Throughout Children's Growth	49
	7.2	Theory of Mind	49
	7.3	Piaget's Theories	50
	7.4	How These Models Can Improve the Dialog with the Child About Illness.	51
		References.	54

Part III Advocates of the Child Who Cannot Speak

8	**The Respect Due and Denied to Those Who Lack Speech**	57
	8.1 The Human Strength of the Speech	57
	8.2 Mentally Impaired Children.	58
	8.3 Perinatal Patients	59
	References.	61
9	**The Communicative Features of Non-verbal Patients.**	63
	9.1 Sensoriality and Pain in the Newborn	63
	9.1.1 Sense Development	63
	9.1.2 The Sense of Pain.	64
	9.2 Communication Skills of the Babies	65
	9.2.1 The Newborn	65
	9.2.2 The Toddler	66
	9.3 Communication Strategies for Mentally Disabled Children	67
	9.3.1 Pain Assessment in Mentally Disabled Children.	70
	9.4 Communicating with Children with Disabilities	70
	9.5 Hearing and Vision Impairment.	73
	References.	73

Part IV What Is a Good Behavior (Aka Ethics)

10 Are You Sure to Know What "Ethics" Really Is? 79
    10.1 Ethics, Virtues, and Protocols 79
          10.1.1 First Premise: The Nonsensical Adjective "Ethical" 79
          10.1.2 Second Premise: Mixing Up Ethics with Rules 80
    10.2 A Synoptic Vision 81
    10.3 Our Ethical Responsibilities 82
    10.4 Children's Ethical Responsibilities 84
    References... 85

11 The Limits of Parental Authority 87
    11.1 Parents Applying Ethical Rules 87
    11.2 End-of-Life Requests...................................... 88
    References... 90

12 To the Depth of Health Care 91
    12.1 The Words That Describe Health Care 91
    12.2 Health: Satisfaction Socially Supported 92
          12.2.1 Health vs. Loneliness in End-of-Life Processes......... 93
    12.3 Supporting Mental Hygiene for a Really Free Choice........... 94
    References... 95

13 Children and Babies: Decisions on Their Health................. 97
    13.1 Treating Every Newborn at All Costs? 97
    13.2 Shifting Too Soon to Palliative Care 99
    13.3 Prejudices Against Disabled Children 99
    References... 100

14 The Pain Principle.. 103
    14.1 Therapeutic Fury 103
    14.2 The Best Interest Principle and Its Limitations 104
    14.3 The Probabilistic Criterion................................. 105
    14.4 The Double Effect 105
    14.5 The Least Harm Criterion 105
    14.6 The Pain Principle 106
    References... 107

Part V The Multiple Approach to Suffering

15 The Environment: The Base of Analgesic Efforts 111
    15.1 Pain Is Not Just "Pain".................................... 111
    15.2 The Hospital as an Analgesic Tool.......................... 112
          15.2.1 Pet-Assisted Therapy 114
          15.2.2 Clown Therapy 114
          15.2.3 Noise-Free Hospital 115
          15.2.4 Meals and Child-Friendly Hospitals.................. 115
    References... 116

16 Assessment of Pain, of Sedation, and of Refractory Symptoms 119
16.1 Pain Assessment 119
16.2 Sedation 122
16.3 Refractory Symptoms 122
References 123

17 Pharmacological and Non-Pharmacological Analgesia 125
17.1 Non-Pharmacological Analgesia 125
    17.1.1 Rhythmic Patterns 126
17.2 Opioids and Other Analgesics 128
    17.2.1 The Earliest Steps of Pharmacological Analgesia 128
    17.2.2 Opioids and Opiates 130
    17.2.3 Main Opioids Used in Pediatrics 131
17.3 Adjuvant Drugs 131
    17.3.1 Steroids 132
    17.3.2 Anticonvulsants 132
    17.3.3 Antidepressants 134
    17.3.4 Neuroleptics 134
    17.3.5 Bisphosphonates and Calcitonin 134
    17.3.6 Placebo 135
    17.3.7 Antineoplastic Drugs 135
    17.3.8 The Conundrum of Cannabinoids 135
    17.3.9 Off-Label Drugs 135
17.4 Sedation 138
References 139

18 Psychological Approach 143
18.1 Meaning-Based Approach 143
18.2 Dignity-Based Approach 144
18.3 Promoting Resilience in Stress Management 145
18.4 Mindfulness 145
References 146

Part VI Palliative Care and Our Fears

19 Children's Pain Scares us 151
19.1 Our Fears 151
19.2 The Three Fearful Paradoxes 152
    19.2.1 Paradox of the Simultaneous Blooming and Dying 152
    19.2.2 Irrational-Reason Paradox 152
    19.2.3 Paradox of the Spectator's Shadow 153
References 155

20 Contagious Pains 157
20.1 Burnout 157
20.2 Overcoming Burnout 159
References 160

21 The Fear of Death and the Errors It Provokes ... 163
21.1 How Fear Can Overshadow Our Judgment ... 163
21.2 Balancing Research and Respect ... 164
References ... 165

22 Overcoming the Fear of Death ... 167
22.1 The Image of Death ... 167
22.2 Rituals ... 168
22.3 Perinatal Mourning ... 169
22.4 Assistance to the Sacredness of Life ... 170
References ... 171

Part VII Types of Pediatric Palliative Care

23 Territorial Differentiation and Home Care ... 175
23.1 The Mission of Pediatric Palliative Care ... 175
23.2 Types of Approach ... 176
23.3 Home Care ... 177
23.4 Community-Based Pediatric Palliative Care ... 178
References ... 180

24 The Pediatric Hospices ... 183
24.1 The Pediatric Hospice ... 183
24.2 Perinatal Hospices ... 184
24.3 Architectural and Structural Guidelines of Pediatric Hospices ... 184
References ... 185

25 Palliative Care Integrated in the Hospital Ward and the Abundance Medicine ... 187
25.1 The Limits of Intensive Set for Palliative Care ... 187
25.2 Pediatric Intensive Care Units: Improvements ... 188
25.3 The Neonatal Intensive Care Unit ... 190
25.4 Parents' Advice ... 190
25.5 Abundance Medicine ... 191
    25.5.1 Healthcare Waste: Defensive Medicine ... 191
    25.5.2 The SUV Effect ... 193
    25.5.3 Abundance Medicine ... 193
References ... 194

26 Conclusion ... 197

Part I
Pediatric Palliative Care: "Fundamentalia"

Without the awareness and knowledge of three important and fundamental assumptions, one cannot think of a well-done pediatric palliative care. The first is the basis of all the basics of medicine: motivation. We will talk about it here with examples and data that leave no doubt that true medical science cannot be practiced if one is not motivated to do so. Then the second fundamental point: understanding what palliative care really is, because it is still thought as a synonym for end-of-life care. This is now an obsolete concept, and to understand it paradoxically we will pass from the history of medicine to the pronouncements of the World Health Organization. Finally, third point: neonatal palliative care. The care of the newborn is different from the care of the older child. This difference is here outlined into three paradoxical phenomena.

This section is fundamental to get good bases and fundaments to build a formidable pediatric palliative care.

The First Obstacle Is in the Handle

1.1 Team-Hierarchy Responsibilities

Everything that will be treated in this book can remain a dead letter: we report here the best practice and the most advanced research in pediatric palliative care, but all these good intentions can rest in a drawer because reading it is just and only the first and merely initial step of improvement. Words and data are useful, but something else comes first. It is like having a sluice that blocks the rushing water of a stream: if you do not open it, the water stagnates, rots, and forms streams and waterfalls that end up elsewhere. The water of the stream is the willpower of doctors and nurses, while the banks of the stream are the guidelines and scientific evidence. But the lock, the "handle," the key, the switch of all this force is those who rule the ward and in the hospital. Has a palliative care center been organized in your hospital? Does it really work? Is there a territorial network of palliative care in your region? And those who manage this center or this network, do they know how to choose the right people? Do they know how to motivate their collaborators?

Hierarchy may seem an obsolete concept in healthcare [1], but hierarchy still has a sense in workload organization and in assumption of responsibilities [2] The main endeavor of the chief of a team or of the hospital is to stay in tune with the proactive and constructive flow of the professionals of that department and to select the most appropriate and motivated personnel. Otherwise, these apical figures can become the above-mentioned sluice, and instead of facilitating health care, they curb it under the burden of protocols and routine.

1.2 Are Doctors Unhappy?

A famous article published a few years ago in the British Medical Journal [3] was entitled: "Why are doctors so unhappy?" and it reads: "The most obvious cause of doctors' unhappiness is that they feel overworked and undersupported. They hear

© The Author(s), under exclusive license to Springer Nature Switzerland AG 2022
C. V. Bellieni, *A New Holistic-Evolutive Approach to Pediatric Palliative Care*, https://doi.org/10.1007/978-3-030-96256-2_1

politicians make extravagant promises but then must explain to patients why the health service cannot deliver what is promised. Endless initiatives are announced, but on the ground, doctors find that operating lists are canceled, they cannot admit or discharge patients, and community services are disappearing. They struggle to respond, but they feel as though they are battling the system rather than being supported by it." But the author added: "And here we come to something deeper—the mismatch between what doctors were trained for and what they are required to do." For example, I add, having transformed the entire relationship of collaboration and trust between doctor and patient into a series of contracts [4, 5] leads to dissatisfaction; the contract is such because it requires you to do what is written even if you would not agree entirely, and it requires you to do nothing more than what is written, even if you would like to be more proactive and more selfless. Is there something that produces more disappointment?

1.3 The Conundrum of Motivation

The US sociologist Berry Schwartz, in his book "Why we Work?" [6] has intelligently taken up this theme, analyzing work in hospitals and other environments and noting widespread dissatisfaction even in the case of increases in incentives and salaries. His diagnosis is that the work often loses its meaning and its taste, and if the work has no taste it becomes boring. And if it gets boring, it leads to medical errors [7].

Now, in current medicine we try to cope with errors by multiplying the defense systems. Reader's criterion of Swiss cheese [8] is well known. According to it, it is necessary to misalign the ways of entry of the error through increasingly refined protocols created to avoid it, as if the ways of entry of the error were the holes inside the Emmental cheese. If we misalign these holes, these channels, the error won't pass. We also know systems that apply corporate criteria to medicine, derived from the assembly line of automobiles, as in the case of the LEAN strategy [9]. These systems suppose that, by multiplying the alerts or by measuring and optimizing production times, it is possible to improve the product, that is, health. But health is not the ratio between costs and benefits [10], between time spent and money saved: it is not a product, but a human feature. Something more is needed. The philosopher Hannah Arendt explained that we put too much of our freedom in the hands of technology. Gunther Anders went so far as to talk about "Promethean envy", reversing the myth of Prometheus, who stole the technique from the gods to bring it to humans (which was called the "Promethean pride"), to be slaves of that technique that we craved so much. Today, we live in a sort of "SUV effect": the SUV is the car so shielded, strong, and protected that it reduces anxiety in the event of an accident, but this paradoxically gets our guard down when, driving. The SUV effect in medicine [4, 5] is the excessive trust we place in the numerous tests we can do and in the numerous drugs we can use, which makes us let our guard down in the face of the disease, thinking that the technique (the tests and the drugs) will do the work for us. But this causes fewer physical visits of patients, less time spent talking to them or, in the case of infants, to their parents [11].

Without syringes, tests cannot be done; but without motivation, the syringes are not used properly, and this increases the risks. The road to follow, then, is that of motivation, to resuscitate medicine and to enter again fresh air in the work of doctors and nurses. But motivation should be favored by the apical figures of healthcare system. A recent study showed that the quality and style of hospital ward supervision is the main factor regulating staff satisfaction [12] And mismanagement or poor governance is the first obstacle to improve healthcare performance [13].

This has an important fallout in pediatric palliative care, where difficult decisions are taken, weak lives are treated and an enormous workload is present. The importance of motivation is here evident, and only people with a deeply ingrained motivation can be effective in working in such a demanding department. Because we cannot hide the core of the problem: being a palliativist exposes to risks for mental balance if not done properly: the acquaintance with death and bereaved parents is devastating and needs to be integrated in a highly motivating environment. However, the path can be simple: the executives satisfy the essential workplace-related needs of medical staff, and healthcare professionals will live and work better, taking care of the reputation of their institution, being more motivated to recognize and satisfy patients' needs. The hospital performance may improve if physicians are wisely and safely guided by their superiors, with motivation, rewards, trainings, and career opportunities [12].

Walker et al. recently described the consequences stress can provoke among surgeons and signaled three levels of action to overcome it: the individual, the team-level, and the institutional ones. *Individual factors* for well-being included autonomy and adequate time to pursue nonclinical endeavors. *Team-level factors* consisted of adaptability, boundaries, and cohesion. *Institutional factors* were related to diversifying performance evaluations and celebrating and recognizing individual value and contributions [14]. Other researchers reported similar results. For instance, Anderson et al. so described the results of a recent analysis performed among New Zealand health professionals: "The three key themes that characterize what matters most to participants' workplace well-being are: a) Supportive team culture b) Delivering excellent patient-centered care, and c) Professional development opportunities. Opportunities to improve well-being also focused on enhancements in these three areas" [15]. It is evident that the first step to get a good feeling in a delicate environment such as pediatric palliative care is a good team, and to get a good team each one's skills and commitments should be exploited and valorized. This is the main role of those responsible for these departments.

Antoine de Saint-Exupéry, author of The Little Prince, illustrated that nicely: "If you want to build a ship, don't drum up the men to gather wood, divide the work and give orders. Instead, teach them to yearn for the vast and endless sea."

This is the first premise for a proactive and smart approach to pediatric and neonatal palliative care: caregivers should be motivated to bear in their minds the supreme interest of their little patients and their families. This motivation should be a continuous endeavor of the department chiefs, so that being empathic and available will not be just a goal, but a prerequisite for physicians and nurses.

References

1. Green B, Oeppen RS, Smith DW, Brennan PA. Challenging hierarchy in healthcare teams—ways to flatten gradients to improve teamwork and patient care. Br J Oral Maxillofac Surg. 2017;55(5):449–53. https://doi.org/10.1016/j.bjoms.2017.02.010. Epub 2017 Mar 23.
2. Wagner C, Mannion R, Hammer A, Groene O, Arah OA, Dersarkissian M, Suñol R, on behalf of the DUQuE Project Consortium. The associations between organizational culture, organizational structure and quality management in European hospitals. Int J Qual Health Care. 2014;26(suppl_1):74–80.
3. Smith R. Why are doctors so unhappy? There are probably many causes, some of them deep. BMJ. 2001;322(7294):1073–74.
4. Bellieni CV. Consumerism: a threat to health? J R Soc Med. 2018a;111(4):112. https://doi.org/10.1177/0141076818763332. Epub 2018 Mar 1.
5. Bellieni CV. Effetto SUV: troppe regole fanno male. La Repubblica; 2018b.
6. Schwartz B. Why we work. Simon & Schuster; 2015.
7. Sung CW, Chen CH, Fan CY, Chang JH, Hung CC, Fu CM, Wong LP, Huang EP, Lee TS. Mental health crisis in healthcare providers in the COVID-19 pandemic: a cross-sectional facility-based survey. BMJ Open. 2021;11(7):e052184. https://doi.org/10.1136/bmjopen-2021-052184.
8. Wiegmann DA, Wood J, L, N Cohen T, Shappell SA. Understanding the "Swiss Cheese Model" and its application to patient safety. J Patient Saf. 2021;18(2):119–23. https://doi.org/10.1097/PTS.0000000000000810.
9. Breen LM, Trepp R Jr, Gavin N. Lean process improvement in the emergency department. Emerg Med Clin North Am. 2020;38(3):633–46. https://doi.org/10.1016/j.emc.2020.05.001. Epub 2020 Jun 11.
10. Steinmann G, van de Bovenkamp H, de Bont A, Delnoij D. Redefining value: a discourse analysis on value-based health care. BMC Health Serv Res. 2020;20(1):862. https://doi.org/10.1186/s12913-020-05614-7.
11. Hershberger PJ, Pei Y, Bricker DA, Crawford TN, Shivakumar A, Vasoya M, Medaramitta R, Rechtin M, Bositty A, Wilson JF. Advancing motivational interviewing training with artificial intelligence: ReadMI. Adv Med Educ Pract. 2021;12:613–8. https://doi.org/10.2147/AMEP.S312373.
12. Chmielewska M, Stokwiszewski J, Filip J, et al. Motivation factors affecting the job attitude of medical doctors and the organizational performance of public hospitals in Warsaw, Poland. BMC Health Serv Res. 2020;20:701. https://doi.org/10.1186/s12913-020-05573-z.
13. Porter ME, Teisberg EO. Redefining health care: creating value-based competition on results. Boston: Harvard Business School Press; 2006.
14. Walker HR, Evans E, Nirula R, Hyngstrom J, Matsen C, Nelson E, Pickron B, Zurbuchen E, Morrow EH. "I need to have a fulfilling job": a qualitative study of surgeon well-being and professional fulfillment. Am J Surg. 2021;223(1):6–11.
15. Anderson N, Pio F, Jones P, Selak V, Tan E, Beck S, Hamilton S, Rogan A, Yates K, Sagarin M, McLeay A, MacLean A, Fayerberg E, Hayward L, Chiang A, Cadzow A, Cadzow N, Moran S, Nicholls M. Facilitators, barriers and opportunities in workplace wellbeing: a national survey of emergency department staff. Int Emerg Nurs. 2021;57:101046. https://doi.org/10.1016/j.ienj.2021.101046. Epub 2021 Jul 6.

Palliative Care Is Not a Synonym of End-of-Life Care

2.1 What Is Palliative Care?

Since its introduction in 1975, the term palliative care has been subject to subtle or substantial changes in meaning [1]. In the long term, the term has been used interchangeably with hospice, end-of-life care, or terminal care [2]. In 1990, the World Health Organization moved away from the equation that used to see palliative care as a synonym for "end of life," stating that palliative care is applicable earlier than at the end of life, that is in the course of the disease, along with cancer treatment or other appropriate therapies [3]. This definition was further changed in 2002, when palliative care was decoupled from prognosis and the target population was expanded to include patients facing a life-threatening condition: "Medicine has always emphasized early recognition of a problem in order to alleviate it or prevent its full development. Similarly, palliative care should be recognized as an exercise in prevention—prevention of ultimate suffering through prioritizing the diagnosis and skillful management of sources of distress, both in the form of physical symptoms and of psychosocial and spiritual concerns, at the earliest possible moment" [4]. The current ideal approach to palliative care, as defined by the World Health Organization, consists in the simultaneous administration of curative and palliative care treatments, with attention to the physical, psychological, social, and spiritual needs of patients. The current definition of palliative care is not limited to what is literally "palliative" ("the alleviation of suffering"), but invokes certain values (such as patient entrality, holism, and multidisciplinarity) that are intended to guide the action and improve clinical practice. The main purpose of palliative care is to maintain the quality and meaningfulness of life for both patients and their families.

Here, it is worth reflecting: the word "palliative" derived from the Latin "pallium" (rag) that signified something that covers and overshadows the sad reality of the end of life. Nowadays, this term "palliative" is obsolete, because this stage of cure is not something useless, or aimed to hide something, but a true branch of medical care. Therefore, when agreeing for palliative care, parents give their consent to the interruption of one type of treatment, but in the perspective of beginning another. It is not the consent to letting die, to giving up, but to continuing the care with adequate though different means of care: what cannot be healed can be cared for.

2.2 Cultural Resistances

In pediatrics and pediatric oncology, early implementation of palliative care has been associated with improved survival and quality of life. According to the document, "Cancer Pain Relief and Palliative Care in Children" [5], pain management for children should begin at the time of diagnosis and continue throughout the course of the disease, along with curative treatments. Despite these recommendations, late referral to the palliativist continues to persist in pediatric oncology [6].

A recent Swiss study conducted among doctors and nurses was carried out in order to evaluate the perception of pediatric palliative care among the treating staff [1]. Most of the participants recognized the important value of pediatric palliative care and had a good understanding of its fundamental principles and objectives. The interesting finding is that, although they clearly distinguished pediatric palliative care from end-of-life or terminal care, many of them insisted that, in the context of pediatric oncology, pediatric palliative care is best prescribed when curative treatment it is no longer an option. Therefore, although WHO guidelines indicate an integrated approach from the time of diagnosis, most participants defined the goal of pediatric palliative care in a much more restrictive sense. However, they also stressed that the transition from curative care to palliative care should not be an abrupt event, but a gradual process during which both families and healthcare professionals - slowly but steadily - become aware of the need to reorient the provision of care. Some participants expressed concern that "mixing" the two care approaches could cause confusion among both family and staff members, and be counterproductive. Confirming the results of previous studies, participants regularly reported difficulties in referring pediatric palliative care services to families, for the strong stigma surrounding the word "palliative". To overcome this obstacle, many participants adopted a euphemistic term, such as "comfort care," "supportive care," or "accompaniment" [1].

2.3 Heterogeneity of Pediatric Cases

When it was first featured in the paper titled "Dying Babies Need Help Too" by Chapman and Goodall [7], pediatric palliative care attracted a lot of attention. In 1998, pediatric palliative care was officially defined as "the active total care of the child's body, mind, and spirit, and involves giving support to the family. It begins when illness is diagnosed and continues regardless of whether or not a child receives treatment directed at the disease" [5] Since 2003, pediatric palliative care has been recognized as a pediatric subspecialty [8] since more and more researchers had noted that children with life-limiting diseases need more attention. In fact, pediatric palliative care is different from palliative care for adults [9], especially in areas such as communication skills with children's parents and bereavement management. It is also different, because the types of diseases, treatments, and care needs vary in different age groups. Furthermore, children without a clear diagnosis are relatively common in pediatric palliative care: in a study performed in 2017, 13.6% of children were without a clear diagnosis at the start of pediatric palliative home care [10]. The unpredictable course of these illnesses has direct implications for palliative care, and the appropriate time to end curative efforts is rarely clearly delineated. This uncertainty is likely to drive much of the delay in initiating palliative services for sick children. Compared to adults with palliative care needs, the group of children is significantly smaller but, at the same time, highly heterogeneous. This heterogeneity concerns: a) the wide age gap from babies, infants, and children to adolescents; b) a broad spectrum of diseases, including rare diseases; c) a variety of needs due to the combination of age, development, and disease, as well as the needs of the whole family [11].

In sum, palliative care for children is an evolving specialty that differs significantly from adult palliative care. Fraser et al. [12] so highlight the main differences:

- The number of children dying is small compared to adults, with many conditions extremely rare and many diagnoses specific to childhood. A recent study showed that children requiring pediatric palliative care in Italy are 34–54 children/100,000 inhabitants, 18/100,000 of whom require specialized pediatric palliative care [13].
- The time scale of children's illnesses differs from that of adults. In children, palliative care may only be needed for a few days, months or, in some cases, it may extend over many years. Life-limiting conditions in children may be familiar; therefore, they may affect more than one child in the family.
- The focus of care is not only the child, but also embraces the whole family. Parents are often expected to become healthcare providers for children with very complex needs, especially those dependent on technology. Pediatric palliative care can offer support in a situation where parents and siblings are particularly vulnerable.
- Despite a diagnosis of a life-limiting condition, children continue to develop physically, emotionally, and cognitively. Of particular interest are the child's communication skills and their ability to understand their condition. Providing education and play when a child is unwell is essential and education is a legal right in many countries.

2.4 The Prophecy of Florence Nightingale

Palliative care is part of a framework of humanization of care and of preventive-social medicine that was pioneered in the last century. We cannot talk about palliative care without reminding that the focus on the influence of the hospital environment on the patient's healing process began with Florence Nightingale, in the nineteenth century. In her book "Notes on Nursing—What is and what is not," she conceptualized the environment as the place where the patient and/or family members are, on a par with their home. Florence Nightingale was an English social reformer, statistician, and the founder of modern nursing. Her first studies were done during the Crimean War in 1915, when she saw that most of the damage to wounded and sick soldiers came from neglect, crowding, lack of hygiene and ventilation of the environment. Speaking of "environment" as fundamental to understanding and treating diseases, she made a great progress in preventive medicine, but she made a further progress by not voluntarily distinguishing between physical, social, and psychological environment: these three components, she said, must be considered interrelated; the key elements of her theory are both the condition and the nature of the patient [14]. Florence Nightingale went further in her analysis: she explained that the key elements for maintaining a healthy environment were ventilation, supply of fresh and pure air, lighting, clarity and direct sunlight, hydration, clothing, play, heat to prevent cooling of patients; but also cleaning for the prevention of infections, avoiding noise, observing silence good smells and food. Furthermore, she included the attention to objects, shapes, and colors to which patients are exposed, as well as the fact that exposure to a positive and clean environment contribute to physical and mental recovery.

Also in her work, she emphasized that children are much more susceptible than adults to harmful influences, that is, they are affected by the same causes, but much more quickly and seriously. To provide adequate care for the child, it is necessary to assure clean air, heat, cleansing the baby's body, room and house, regular food, bright and cheerful environment, appropriate bedding and personal clothing. And she pointed out the importance of neither scaring the babies nor stressing them [14].

It is worth remembering that the scenario indicated by Florence Nightingale in her theory is the domestic environment, however in her work "Notes on hospitals," published in 1863 [15], she prescribes the principles for the construction of hospitals, having harmony as a reference between environment and construction technique. Among the principles, the orientation of the building with respect to the sun is highlighted; she also gave references about the exposure to prevailing winds, size and positioning of windows and doors, thermal resistance of walls and roofs, as well as an optimal performance in terms of energy efficiency through the horizontality of the buildings called "Pavilion." (so called for their shape similar to a butterfly, "papillon" in French).

The attention to the environment she claimed, is reflected in the principles of today's humanized care, based on the control of the environment around the patients, who relay and interact with the environment in which they are inserted. Florence Nightingale's thought has a primary influence on the professional modern nursing, leading the reflection to the current ecological problems linked to the combination of health and the environment.

This is now an ancient reflection; however, it is topical for the units that serve the pediatric age: it is a priority to provide a stimulating environment, suitable for the different phases of the child's growth and development, to provide a more effective recovery through a less traumatic hospitalization for the children and their families.

It is also topical for hospices and intensive care units: the best standards for child-friendly and family-friendly hospitality have still these bases.

References

1. De Clercq E, Rost M, Rakic M, et al. The conceptual understanding of pediatric palliative care: a Swiss healthcare perspective. BMC Palliat Care. 2019;18:55.
2. Foster T. Pediatric palliative care revisited. A vision to add life. J Hosp Palliat Nurs. 2007;9:212–9.
3. World Health Organization. Definition of palliative care. https://www.who.int/cancer/palliative/definition/en/.
4. World Health Organization. National cancer control programmes: policies and managerial guidelines. 2nd ed. Geneva: World Health Organization; 2002.
5. World Health Organization. Cancer pain relief and palliative care in children. Geneva: WHO; 1998.
6. Zhen ZJ, Sun XF, Xia Y, Ling JY, Zheng L, Luo WB, Lin H. [Feasibility to treat pediatric cancer pain with analgesics for adults and their efficacy]. Ai Zheng. 2007;26(8):866–869.
7. Chapmn JA, Goodall J. Dying children need help too. Br Med J. 1979;1:593–4.
8. Hutchinson F. Terminal care in paediatrics: where we are now. Postgrad Med. 2003;79(936):566e8.
9. Zhang M, Li X. Focuses and trends of the studies on pediatric palliative care: a bibliometric analysis from 2004 to 2018. Int J Nurs Sci. 2020;8(1):5–14.
10. Hoell JI, Warfsmann J, Gagnon G, Trocan L, Balzer S, Oommen PT, et al. Palliative care for children with a yet undiagnosed syndrome. Eur J Pediatr. 2017;176(10):1319e27.
11. Bergstr€asser E. Paediatric Palliative Care: what is different in children compared to adults? Ther Umschau Revue Ther. 2018;75(2):101e4.
12. Fraser LK, Bluebond-Langner M, Ling J. Advances and challenges in European Paediatric Palliative Care. Med Sci (Basel). 2020;8(2):20. https://doi.org/10.3390/medsci8020020.
13. Benini F, Bellentani M, Reali L, Lazzarin P, De Zen L, Pellegatta F, Aprile PL, Scaccabarozzi G. An estimation of the number of children requiring pediatric palliative care in Italy. Ital J Pediatr. 2021;47(1):4. https://doi.org/10.1186/s13052-020-00952-y.
14. Nightingale F. Florence nightingale and the war. Hospital (Lond 1886). 1916;59(1550):487–8.
15. Nightingale F. Notes on hospitals. Dover Pubns; 2015. Reprint edizione.

Neonatal and Perinatal Care

3

3.1 Three Paradoxes

We should not neglect a peculiar part of pediatric palliative care: neonatal care. Neonatology is an important part of pediatrics; therefore, the general lines and data that we will bring about pediatric palliative care are valid here as well; but the newborn has a peculiar world. Newborns are fragile, they do not speak, they do not even communicate satisfaction or sorrow through their behavior that is not yet structured and explicit. They must be deciphered in their signals and movements or in their silences. But above all, neonatal palliative care has three typical features, that are the paradoxes of sick newborns, and that astonish the unexperienced caregiver.

3.1.1 First Paradox: Little Bodies Do Not Mean Little Grief

The first paradox is that parents' grief for a newborn happens in a particular phase of the emotional development and attachment of their parents: the attachment parents have for their 10-year-old child is different from that for a 10-day-old baby. It is natural: the family gets structured little by little, as affection and attachment grow. But this does not mean that the grief for the loss or the pain of a future disability will be lower; they are just different, or even greater [1]. Because one feeling (grief) is being elaborated by parents simultaneously with another one (attachment), which normally acts as a substrate and support for the former. Usually, grief and attachment happen in two distinct periods of the life; in the case of sick newborns, they are overlapped and confused, and this leads to a great existential confusion. In fact, every feeling one has for a person or for an object depends on how much one has invested on them; but here parents had no time for this investment, and it is still in progress.

© The Author(s), under exclusive license to Springer Nature Switzerland AG 2022
C. V. Bellieni, *A New Holistic-Evolutive Approach to Pediatric Palliative Care*, https://doi.org/10.1007/978-3-030-96256-2_3

Thus, a myth should be demystified. It may seem that the level of feelings experienced by parents about the newborns' disease or death must be low because their affective investment is not yet fully developed. Instead, the opposite happens: in the first moments after birth there is a very strong affective-hormonal charge [2] that is not yet a peaceful and daily attachment, but that is giving the energy to get it. It is like when you are igniting a car to get a high cruising speed: the first kilometers you drive to put it into the race are more expensive for the engine than when you have reached the desired speed, because the first kilometers were run at an obviously lower yet more intense speed. This phenomenon has recently been studied by De Marchi et al., who have shown how the presence of high levels of oxytocin in the blood of the woman, who has recently given birth, conflict with a mourning, leading to a high risk of mental sequelae [3]. So, what happens - good or bad - during the period of ongoing attachment, happens in a period of intense feelings, troubles, and emotions, and its consequences are extreme. In fact, in the event of an unfortunate outcome, psychological dramas occur, mental dilemmas are not solved, and parental couples often separate [4].

3.1.2 Second Paradox: Little Bodies Do Not Mean Little Pain

The second characteristic is that newborns feel pain exactly like adults [5]; perhaps more than adults, according to what Rebecca Slater reports, speaking about her study on neonatal pain (https://www.ox.ac.uk/news/2015-04-2-babies-feel-pain-adults). It seems counter-intuitive, because a small body and a small brain seem necessarily produce a small pain. However, it is the opposite: the newborn's nervous system has well-developed paths for pain, but it has not yet developed the ways to inhibit it [6, 7]. So, the pain that the little patient feels is more intense, less defined, and probably even more distressing (the amygdala, center of stress analysis, is already active in the newborn). Unfortunately, the hospitalized severely sick newborn undergoes more than 15 painful events per day, 80% of which without specific analgesia [8]; this would be unacceptable for older children. They do not even have the support of their parents, sometimes because they are not present at the time of the maneuvers, sometimes because parents do not realize if the movements that the newborn makes are due to pain or are quite physiological [9]. The first cause of this mistreatment is this never-ending prejudice: "the smaller the baby, the lower the pain." In fact, though the neonatal intensive care environment is a frantic environment, full of noises, lights and overcrowded, newborns in their incubators undergo noises, shocks, and bangs [10] that are not acknowledged from the outside, simply because none dares to put themselves in neonates' shoes, as babies seem so "different" and so small.

Nonetheless, most of the pain-relieving drugs that we will discuss in the text are available for the newborn, even though many of them are used off-label [11], and others are almost contraindicated (opioids can damage the brain of the newborn who will survive [12], and therefore they should be used smartly). Thus, the way of relieving and preventing their pain would be available, as well as the prevention of the sources of stress.

3.1.3 Third Paradox: Small Age Does Not Mean Small Rights

The third feature is newborn's viability and its consequences on care. Viability means a child's ability to survive, helped by the medical commitment. Viability has a limit: sometimes the babies must undergo compassionate end-of-life treatments, because there is no reasonable hope of survival for them for example, if a fetus is born prematurely at 20–22 weeks of gestation: its alveoli are not still effective, and every attempt to give oxygen to the blood is useless. Obviously, this age limit has moved back with the progress of medicine [13]. Ten years ago, it would have been said that the limit was 24 weeks, and 40 years ago it was 26 weeks. For some protocols, there is a period in which survival is not impossible but neither guaranteed, and it is defined a "gray" period, in which one may or may not actively resuscitate these children [14] with different criteria from one country to another [15]. Now some centers report that more than half of babies born at 22 weeks survive and most survivors are neurocognitively intact or do not have severe pathologies. Yet, many centers do not offer life-sustaining treatment to babies born so prematurely [16]. The gray zone is not only referred to survival; it is also that one that follows a prognosis of incertitude on the future integrity of the baby [17]. The consequence is that children who are in this gray limbo can receive either intensive care or only palliative care. The choice between these two possibilities is often subjective, with different protocols that suggest different decisions for these babies. Paradoxically, this gray-zone criterion with decisions taken on the basis of the possible future disability is not used for older children or adults [18]; this difference in treatment has raised great perplexity in many [19], raising the hypothesis of discrimination against the infants [20]. Babies can risk severe anoxic brain damage after birth or can have chromosomal abnormalities diagnosed before birth, and some clinics actively assist them and others do not, often based on the desire or decision of their parents rather than on the pure prognosis [21]. For example, trisomies 13 and 18 are two cases of diseases that get compassionate treatment and no active treatment in many countries [22], though the cases in which these children are also treated surgically to correct some of their problems are more and more frequent [23]. Another example is the hypoplasia of the left heart, which was once thought not to leave chance to the children [24] and directed them, when it was available, to palliative care; nowadays, an active approach is increasingly used [25]. The better prognosis in these cases is due to not having given up hope and having made some centers try to cure this disease.

On this point, Keith Barrington, neonatologist and bioethicist so wrote: "Many ethicists have proposed that in order to consider redirection of care to comfort care rather than curative care, the mayor consideration should be: should this patient have a potential for a good quality of life or not? There is one test we can indeed use to predict future quality of life in the extremely preterm infant at discharge from hospital. The test is simple: 'Is the baby alive?' If the answer is yes, the positive predictive value for an acceptable to excellent quality of life is 95%" [26].

3.2 Perinatal Palliative Care

Current medicine can cure some prenatally diagnosed diseases, for example, with prenatal surgery, or can make a diagnosis with fetal ultrasound and prepare to treat the fetus at birth. Unfortunately, sometimes there are no therapies to heal the fetus. Some diseases are so serious that they leave no hope [27, 28]: the fetus will be born and will die in a few days. Hence, the importance of perinatal palliative care. Perinatal palliative care has a particular approach: it takes care of the parents up to birth, and of both the newborn and their parents thereafter.

This type of treatment has three stages. The first stage is the communication with the parents, that often is a step within prenatal diagnosis. The second stage is the preparation to the birth. The third stage is the environmental and pharmacological palliative care to be performed after birth. All these stages are integrative parts of palliative care, including those of communication and preparation to birth.

First stage. Communicating a life-threatening condition to the parents is traumatic [29]. Perhaps there is no greater pain which can be given to a mother and father. But in this case, the fetuses that die are not yet fully present: *it* is there but cannot be seen or touched. So, parents, when being informed of the terminal state of their fetus, start their grief for a baby who still does not look like a baby [30]. This is bewildering. In the case of a newborn, parents have a physical body in their hands, and even their attachment process is tumultuously beginning and ending, with the risks we have illustrated; but here, int the case of fetal death or severe disease, they experience an even worse contradiction: elaborating a grief when they are not yet elaborating attachment. Grief triggers and threatens their attachment in an unnatural way during the process of elaboration of the mother-baby symbiosis, when the symbiosis is not yet mature, and when that mother-baby couple [31, 32] that creates the new life of the mother and the new life of the child has not been constituted yet, another elaboration improperly begins: grief [33]. It is as if shipwrecked people see the beach for a moment, but it suddenly disappears. They cannot weep without a body, to which offer pain, love, contact, farewell. So, depression and guilt are fierce, and ready to attack both mom and dad. Therefore, it is necessary to help parents even before the birth of their baby; there must be a structured path for these cases, in which a team made of different specialists accompany the parents in the knowledge of their baby's disease and in processing their grief [34]. The prenatal phase of perinatal care is not just diagnosis and communication, but it features other two points: (a) submitting an opportune path of specialists for that specific case to the parents: the gynecologist cannot be an "all-rounder"; (b) offering parents a psychological help in the provision of birth.

The second stage is birth. In these cases, the child must be born in a center equipped to provide confirmation or disconfirmation of the prenatal disease and its severity, and to provide the opportune treatments. Then, it must be able to provide the appropriate reserved and welcoming environment for the baby and their family.

The third stage is providing assistance in the last days or weeks of life to the child and their family. For this reason, special prenatal hospices have been created in various centers: places different from the common ward of the hospital, where the family is housed and cared for throughout these days [35]. And here all the tools of good palliative care should be used: painkillers, nutrition, and psychological, religious, and family support [36, 37]. Lastly, we must not forget the importance of the images, of the memories, of the little things that the baby touched, small traces for the elaboration of the grief; as well as the importance of the wake, the funeral, the burial, and of the tomb, a place where parents can remember it and, if necessary, weep.

References

1. Institute of Medicine (US) Committee on Palliative and End-of-Life Care for Children and Their Families; Field MJ, Behrman RE, editors. When children die: improving palliative and end-of-life care for children and their families. Washington (DC): National Academies Press (US); 2003. APPENDIX E, BEREAVEMENT EXPERIENCES AFTER THE DEATH OF A CHILD. https://www.ncbi.nlm.nih.gov/books/NBK220798/
2. Kirsch M, Buchholz MB. On the nature of the mother-infant tie and its interaction with Freudian drives. Front Psychol. 2020;11:317. https://doi.org/10.3389/fpsyg.2020.00317.
3. Demarchi L, Pawluski JL, Bosch OJ. The brain oxytocin and corticotropin-releasing factor systems in grieving mothers: what we know and what we need to learn. Peptides. 2021;143:170593. https://doi.org/10.1016/j.peptides.2021.170593. Epub 2021 Jun 6.
4. Torkild Hovde Lyngstad. Bereavement and divorce: does the death of a child affect parents' marital stability? Family Science. 2013;4(1):79–86.
5. Goksan S, Hartley C, Emery F, Cockrill N, Poorun R, Moultrie F, Rogers R, Campbell J, Sanders M, Adams E, Clare S, Jenkinson M, Tracey I, Slater R. fMRI reveals neural activity overlap between adult and infant pain. elife. 2015;4:e06356. https://doi.org/10.7554/eLife.06356. Erratum in: Elife. 2015;4. doi: 10.7554/eLife.08663.
6. Chau CMY, Ranger M, Bichin M, Park MTM, Amaral RSC, Chakravarty M, Poskitt K, Synnes AR, Miller SP, Grunau RE. Hippocampus, amygdala, and thalamus volumes in very preterm children at 8 years: neonatal pain and genetic variation. Front Behav Neurosci. 2019;13:51. https://doi.org/10.3389/fnbeh.2019.00051.
7. Goksan S, Baxter L, Moultrie F, Duff E, Hathway G, Hartley C, Tracey I, Slater R. The influence of the descending pain modulatory system on infant pain-related brain activity. elife. 2018;7:e37125. https://doi.org/10.7554/eLife.37125.
8. Carbajal R, Rousset A, Danan C, Coquery S, Nolent P, Ducrocq S, Saizou C, Lapillonne A, Granier M, Durand P, Lenclen R, Coursol A, Hubert P, de Saint BL, Boëlle PY, Annequin D, Cimerman P, Anand KJ, Bréart G. Epidemiology and treatment of painful procedures in neonates in intensive care units. JAMA. 2008;300(1):60–70. https://doi.org/10.1001/jama.300.1.60.
9. Palomaa AK, Korhonen A, Pölkki T. Factors Influencing Parental Participation in Neonatal Pain Alleviation. J Pediatr Nurs. 2016;31(5):519–27.
10. Bellieni CV, Buonocore G, Pinto I, Stacchini N, Cordelli DM, Bagnoli F. Use of sound-absorbing panel to reduce noisy incubator reverberating effects. Biol Neonate. 2003;84(4):293–6. https://doi.org/10.1159/000073637.
11. Tesoro S, Marchesini V, Fratini G, Engelhardt T, De Robertis E. Drugs for anesthesia and analgesia in the preterm infant. Minerva Anestesiol. 2020;86(7):742–55. https://doi.org/10.23736/S0375-9393.20.14073-2. Epub 2020 Jan 28.
12. Alipio JB, Haga C, Fox ME, Arakawa K, Balaji R, Cramer N, Lobo MK, Keller A. Perinatal fentanyl exposure leads to long-lasting impairments in somatosensory circuit function and behavior. J Neurosci. 2021;41(15):3400–17. https://doi.org/10.1523/JNEUROSCI.2470-20.2021.

13. Di Stefano LM, Wood K, Mactier H, Bates SE, Wilkinson D. Viability and thresholds for treatment of extremely preterm infants: survey of UK neonatal professionals. Arch Dis Child Fetal Neonatal Ed. 2021;106(6):596–602. https://doi.org/10.1136/archdischild-2020-321273. Epub ahead of print.
14. Wilkinson AR, Ahluwalia J, Cole A, Crawford D, Fyle J, Gordon A, Moorcraft J, Pollard T, Roberts T. Management of babies born extremely preterm at less than 26 weeks of gestation: a framework for clinical practice at the time of birth. Arch Dis Child Fetal Neonatal Ed. 2009;94(1):F2–5. https://doi.org/10.1136/adc.2008.143321. Epub 2008 Oct 6.
15. Lantos JD, Meadow W. Variation in the treatment of infants born at the borderline of viability. Pediatrics. 2009;123(6):1588–90. https://doi.org/10.1542/peds.2009-0030.
16. Lantos JD. Ethical issues in treatment of babies born at 22 weeks of gestation. Arch Dis Child. 2021;106(12):1155–7. https://doi.org/10.1136/archdischild-2020-320871. Epub ahead of print.
17. Stolz E, Burkert N, Großschädl F, Rásky É, Stronegger WJ, Freidl W. Determinants of public attitudes towards euthanasia in adults and physician-assisted death in neonates in Austria: a national survey. PLoS One. 2015;10(4):e0124320. https://doi.org/10.1371/journal.pone.0124320.
18. Janvier A, Barrington KJ, Aziz K, Bancalari E, Batton D, Bellieni C, Bensouda B, Blanco C, Cheung PY, Cohn F, Daboval T, Davis P, Dempsey E, Dupont-Thibodeau A, Ferretti E, Farlow B, Fontana M, Fortin-Pellerin E, Goldberg A, Hansen TW, Haward M, Kovacs L, Lapointe A, Lantos J, Morley C, Moussa A, Musante G, Nadeau S, O'Donnell CP, Orfali K, Payot A, Ryan CA, Sant'anna G, Saugstad OD, Sayeed S, Stokes TA, Verhagen E. CPS position statement for prenatal counselling before a premature birth: simple rules for complicated decisions. Paediatr Child Health. 2014;19(1):22–4.
19. Janvier A, Lantos J, Deschênes M, Couture E, Nadeau S, Barrington KJ. Caregivers attitudes for very premature infants: what if they knew? Acta Paediatr. 2008;97(3):276–9. https://doi.org/10.1111/j.1651-2227.2008.00663.x.
20. Bellieni CV, Tei M, Coccina F, Buonocore G. Why do we treat the newborn differently? J Matern Fetal Neonatal Med. 2012;25(Suppl 1):73–5. https://doi.org/10.3109/14767058.2012.663178. Epub 2012 Mar 8.
21. Kunz SN, McAdams RM, Diekema DS, Opel DJ. A quality of life quandary: a framework for navigating parental refusal of treatment for co-morbidities in infants with underlying medical conditions. J Clin Ethics. 2015;26(1):16–23.
22. Pyle AK, Fleischman AR, Hardart G, et al. Management options and parental voice in the treatment of trisomy 13 and 18. J Perinatol. 2018;38:1135–43.
23. Weaver MS, Lantos J, Hauschild K, Hammel J, Birge N, Janvier A. Communicating with parents of children with trisomy 13 or 18 who seek cardiac interventions. Cardiol Young. 2021;31(3):471–5. https://doi.org/10.1017/S1047951120004023. Epub 2020 Nov 19
24. Norwood WI. Hypoplastic left heart syndrome. Cardiol Clin. 1989;7(2):377–85.
25. Palacios-Macedo A, Díliz-Nava H, García-Benítez L, Pérez-Juárez F, Tamariz-Cruz O. Norwood procedure in a patient with hypoplastic left heart syndrome, right aortic arch, and right descending aorta. World J Pediatr Congenit Heart Surg. 2021;12(5):682–4. https://doi.org/10.1177/21501351211027856. Epub ahead of print.
26. Barrington K. Predicting outcomes in the very preterm infant. In: Verhagen E, Janvier A, editors. Ethical dilemmas for critically ill babies. Springer; 2016.
27. Lynser D, Marbaniang E. Sonographic images of fetal terminal myelocystocele: a rare form of closed spinal dysraphism. Acta Neurol Belg. 2016;116(2):199–200. https://doi.org/10.1007/s13760-015-0539-4. Epub 2015 Sep 10.
28. Syngelaki A, Hammami A, Bower S, Zidere V, Akolekar R, Nicolaides KH. Diagnosis of fetal non-chromosomal abnormalities on routine ultrasound examination at 11-13 weeks' gestation. Ultrasound Obstet Gynecol. 2019;54(4):468–76. https://doi.org/10.1002/uog.20844.
29. Kratovil AL, Julion WA. Health-care provider communication with expectant parents during a prenatal diagnosis: an integrative review. J Perinatol. 2017;37(1):2–12. https://doi.org/10.1038/jp.2016.123. Epub 2016 Aug 11.

References

30. Serra G, Memo L, Coscia A, Giuffré M, Iuculano A, Lanna M, Valentini D, Contardi A, Filippeschi S, Frusca T, Mosca F, Ramenghi LA, Romano C, Scopinaro A, Villani A, Zampino G, Corsello G, their respective Scientific Societies and Parents' Associations. Recommendations for neonatologists and pediatricians working in first level birthing centers on the first communication of genetic disease and malformation syndrome diagnosis: consensus issued by 6 Italian scientific societies and 4 parents' associations. Ital J Pediatr. 2021;47(1):94. https://doi.org/10.1186/s13052-021-01044-1.
31. Croughs W. De vroege ouder-kindrelatie [The early parent-child relationship]. Tijdschr indergeneeskd. 1984;52(2):39–49.
32. Resta G. Gravidanza e allattamento al seno: stadi evolutivi della coppia madre-figlio [Pregnancy and breast-feeding: developmental stages of mother-child bonding]. Ann Ostet Ginecol Med Perinat. 1992;113(4):201–6.
33. Boss RD. Building relationships in the neonatal intensive care unit to improve infant outcomes. Patient Educ Couns. 2021;104(7):1503–4. https://doi.org/10.1016/j.pec.2021.05.004.
34. Lou S, Petersen OB, Lomborg K, Vogel I. How do geneticists and prospective parents interpret and negotiate an uncertain prenatal genetic result? An analysis of clinical interactions. J Genet Couns. 2020;29(6):1221–33. https://doi.org/10.1002/jgc4.1290. Epub 2020 May 26.
35. Korzeniewska-Eksterowicz A, Kozinska J, Kozinski K, Dryja U. Prenatal diagnosis of a lethal defect: what next? History of first family in perinatal hospice. Palliat Support Care. 2021:1–2. https://doi.org/10.1017/S1478951521000870. Epub ahead of print.
36. Qian J, Sun S, Wu M, Liu L, Yaping S, Yu X. Preparing nurses and midwives to provide perinatal bereavement care: a systematic scoping review. Nurse Educ Today. 2021;103:104962. https://doi.org/10.1016/j.nedt.2021.104962. Epub 2021 May 18.
37. Benini F, Congedi S, Rusalen F, Cavicchiolo ME, Lago P. Barriers to perinatal palliative care consultation. Front Pediatr. 2020;8:590616. https://doi.org/10.3389/fped.2020.590616.

Part II

Communication with Children and Their Families

In this section, we deal with the theme of communication with children and their family. It is divided into various parts to highlight various aspects of communication: adapting the communication to the age of the child, the character of the child and the family, and to the stage of their grief. All this is not meant to be an instruction for the use of words, attitudes, and situations, but an encouragement to a synoptic vision, that is, a vision that gives an overview of the situation and at the same time collaborates makes the caregiver able to collaborate with the patient throughout their development of bereavement and growth. On the converse, applying only rules in the communication field, communicates a sad lack of spontaneity. We need to educate ourselves to familiarity with the patient: this is the first step for a true communication. All the details described here will be useful embankments and signs to learn how to encounter our patient and to take care of their global health.

Words Can Break My Heart

4.1 Crucial Importance of the Interview

Communicating is a basic point of palliative care. We are dealing with difficult, painful, tiring, tragic, exhausting things and the words we use are a real therapy; or a lethal weapon.

Before learning "how" to communicate, we must become aware of one crucial matter: you communicate only if you and your patient are on the same wavelength. The verb "to communicate" is derived from Latin and it means "to bear together a duty" (from the words "cum" that means "with" and "munus" that means "duty"); so that it is a reciprocal and solidaristic action, that requires three standing points:

1. being companions and not counterparts of those who stand in front of us
2. allow a relationship gap to stand between the two: an excessive closeness is negative
3. never let those with whom we are communicating think that we are following a protocol and a manual on how to speak with them [1]

In short, to talk about death, we must be concerned with life: caring for the life of the person in front of us, and not being scared by their death. It is a paradox, and we will find many in this book dealing with a destructuring, disrupting but also creative matter. It is hard to simultaneously speak professionally and wholeheartedly, but sometimes it is better to avoid talking if we risk to seem cold, abrupt, and careless [2].

The interview between doctor and family, or doctor and child, should not only be useful for those who receive the information, but also for those who provide it can seem that only someone talks and someone else only listens, but it is a two-way process; both doctor and patient will be humanly enriched if silence, time, and postures were used to confront not two people united by a contract, an operator, and a client, but two human beings. And while the patient gets informed, the doctor acquires new details and sees new aspects of the whole story. The encounter of two humanities is always fruitful [3, 4].

Nonetheless, in receiving bad news a complex interaction starts. Sorrow and anxiety become contagious, an interaction of suspects and diffidence can be unleashed. Moreover, parents may make believe to be serene in order to not anguish the child and vice versa [5] and this can be a real obstacle, as we will see later. So, experience is important in these moments, as well as the ability to remain calm and professional despite the disappointment.

4.2 The False Myth of Empathy

Minors cannot decide; they can listen and speak, but it is their parents who decide. Nonetheless, it is a false belief thinking that since the children do not decide, it is not worth talking to them. Minors can give a consent to their care, though incomplete, because care can only be authorized by those who have an effective decision-making authority, that is, their parents, or in some cases the minor's guardian, and only on behalf of and in the interest of the minor [6, 7]. But this parental process passes through the dialog with the child, if this is possible. Recommendations have been developed to help deliver bad news to the parents and adult patients, while less clear are the recommendations on how to communicate the diagnosis directly to the children. So, direct communication with these little patients is sometimes avoided, in part for fear of how the child will react [8], in part because we think it is useless; this communication is demanded to the child's family and this is often a mistake: children, their families, and the doctors are a small community [9] despite the difference of their roles.

One recommendation is here noteworthy: do not transform empathy into a myth. Empathy is important in the dialog with the children or their families, but it is only a part of the matter. The dialog with the children and families is mutual and based on reciprocity, but the two actors (doctor and patient) are not equivalent: doctors know many things that patients ignore and vice versa, and both should offer their experience remaining in their own range. Moreover, empathy has the limit of an insuperable fence: children's deep secret area that sometimes is unknown to parents and sometimes to the children themselves. It is a sacred, inviolable area of thoughts, beliefs, hates and fears that you cannot dare enter in (Fig. 4.1). Therefore, the dialog cannot have the utopian myth of open knowledge or of persuading with the speech; persuasion happens through acts, through what is seen or perceived. The bad news is that words are weak in exorting children to make their best interest; the good news is that most of the job is done by our being present, and perceived as sincere, available, and professional.

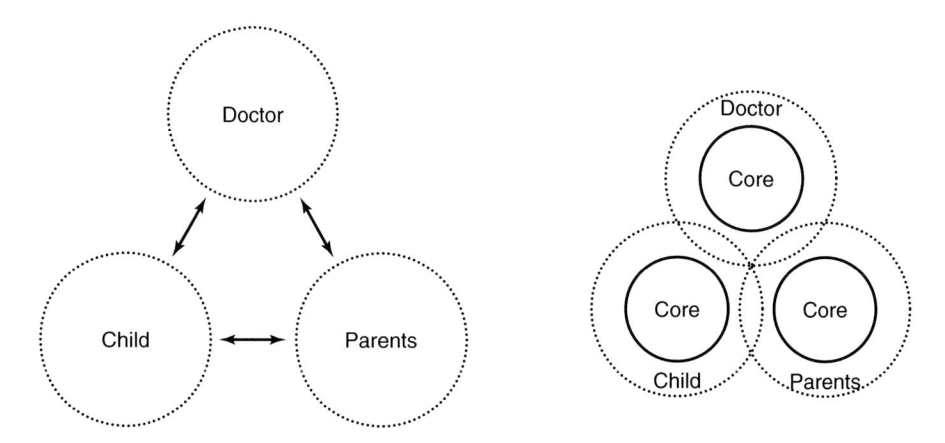

Fig. 4.1 Empathy. The common relationship among doctors, children, and parents is illustrated in the figure on the left, where a distance between all these actors in maintained. The concept of empathy tightens the relationships, though maintaining an individual sacredness, the "core" of any actor

4.3 Certain News Is Indelible

It marks, it scares: it is the moment when the diagnosis is disclosed; it will be vividly remembered for many years, and signs the beginning of a new journey for the family.

The doctor in those moments and in those cases is not just a provider of information, as if they had a manual with the instructions for the treatment or a leaflet with the prognosis. Doctors are someone whose words and silences and data will reshape the family, so errors in this step will leave wounds that hurt, that bleed [10].

What does "errors" mean here? It is not a matter of "what," it is a matter of "how."

A colloquium is not only the use of words, but time, space, smiles. You cannot speak "as I would like to be addressed in similar situations" or as if you were following a protocol, because protocols and manuals are essential to fix and repair a car, but not in human relationships. Unfortunately, much of what is learnt in Medical Schools is following protocols, and this is one of the more evident causes of sanitary dissatisfaction, because just following protocols at most leads to mediocrity [11]. And in this scenario, this is utterly evident.

Giving the consent to palliative care is not just giving the consent to new treatments, as it usually happens. In most cases, it is a drama, as it means becoming aware that life-saving therapies have failed. It means to allow withdrawing the therapies the patient was receiving in the hope of recovery, it means giving the consent to move towards a terminal phase, accepting that the hopes of recovery are gone.

But this also means starting an alternative therapeutic path, because palliative care is not only a way of masking death with a rag to cover up the pain and sadness of the last days: it is an active, useful scientific treatment [12]. Thus, patients have to be approached in this moment with care and attention, they should have all the time they need to discuss, to reflect and decide on the different options that palliative care offers.

4.3.1 Silence

The interview is not just words, but also movements, gestures, times, and silences. In some cases, silences are more important than words. Silence must be respected and must be deepened. Silence is not an absence, but an instrument of communication within the "therapeutic listening" [13]. Often, we think that only what we do is useful, and what we say is the only understandable matter; but what we do not do an also be very useful, as well as what we do not say. Silence takes the largest and most relevant part of the time we spend doing something, because our acts are made of pauses, reflections, silences, scares, uncertainties; and it is through these pauses that the patient can explore our reliability and our availability [14].

We must not be afraid of silence, an integrant part of the speech; we should not fill it with inopportune words. Through pauses it is possible to give a complete information to a minor who, as we will see, seldom cannot be involved into a colloquium as an adult. Being silent, if necessary, is important, without being scared by it, because some silences are more eloquent than many words [15].

4.3.2 The Informed Consent

The "informed consent" is important to guarantee the patient's rights, but sometimes it is something just aimed to guarantee the doctor's acts. The real meaning of the informed consent should be questioned and challenged because someone may think it is just a series of signatures we need from the parents in order to do some interventions. This has two main causes: first, our desire that after the signature, our commitment be over, and - if the patient has chosen something we disapprove-, we may think that the consequences are not our matter; second, that in our minds the informed consent can have not the aim of allowing patients to make a careful choice, but just that of preserving us from complains. This is unacceptable. The informed consent is not just a paper to sign, but it is a process of knowledge and awareness that requires time, dialog, acquaintainceship, disponibility, and silence; the signature, as well as the paper to sign, is just the final action in a path. Anyway, the paper to sign, that should only be the summary of the above process, should not be unreadable or extremely redundant, as it often happens [16]. Avoid paternalism: according to some philosophers [17], the concept of "consent" is connected to a passive behavior and should be replaced by that of "request," where well-informed patients ask a type of treatment after several specialistic consultations, and their endeavor is not limited to accepting or refusing what is proposed to them. This can have several drawbacks, in particular in the Google-era, when the availability of medical information is huge and sometimes misleading. It is worth remembering what Jay Katz wrote in 1994: "Nuland [a surgeon, author of the Book "How we Die"] pleads for the resurrection of the family doctor because he believes that the specialist is inadequate to the task of shouldering the burdens of decision with his patients. About this I differ with him. I believe that physicians (and surgeons as well) can, and must, learn to converse with patients in the spirit of joint decision-making. Physicians can and must learn to appreciate better than they do now that the principle of respect for person speaks to the caring commitment of physicians in old and new ways: Old in that it highlights the ancient and venerable medical duty not to abandon patients, and new by requiring doctors to communicate with them and remain at their sides, not only while their bodies are racked with pain and suffering but also while their minds are beset by fear, confusion, doubt and suffering over decisions to be made; also new in that implementation of the principle of psychological autonomy imposes the obligations on physicians both to invite, and respond to, questions about the decisions to be made, and to do so by respecting patients' ultimate choices, a new aspect of the duty to care" [18].

References

1. Martino R. El proceso de morir en el nino y en el adolescente. Pediatr Integral. 2007;12:926–34.
2. Melin-Johansson C, Axelsson I, Jonsson Grundberg M, Hallqvist F. When a child dies: parents' experiences of palliative care-an integrative literature review. J Pediatr Nurs. 2014;29(6):660–9. https://doi.org/10.1016/j.pedn.2014.06.009. Epub 2014 Jun 26.
3. Cao EL, Blinderman CD, Cross I. Reconsidering empathy: an interpersonal approach and participatory arts in the medical humanities. J Med Humanit. 2021;42(4):627–40. https://doi.org/10.1007/s10912-021-09701-6. Epub ahead of print.
4. Yu W, Chen J, Sun S, Liu P, Ouyang L, Hu J. The reciprocal associations between caregiver burden, and mental health in primary caregivers of cancer patients: a longitudinal study: family functioning, caregiver burden, and mental health Wenjun Yu et al. Psychooncology. 2021;30(6):892–900. https://doi.org/10.1002/pon.5667. Epub 2021 Mar 9.
5. Hrdlickova L, Polakova K, Loucka M. Important aspects influencing delivery of serious news in pediatric oncology: a scoping review. Children (Basel). 2021;8(2):166. https://doi.org/10.3390/children8020166.
6. Hickey K. Minors' rights in medical decision making. JONAS Healthc Law Ethics Regul. 2007;9(3):100–4.
7. Wilson EH, Burkle CM. The meaning of consent and its implications for anesthesiologists. Adv Anesth. 2020;38:1–22. https://doi.org/10.1016/j.aan.2020.07.001. Epub 2020 Aug 14.
8. Bradford N, Rolfe M, Ekberg S, Mitchell G, Beane T, Ferranti K, Herbert A. Family meetings in paediatric palliative care: an integrative review. BMJ Support Palliat Care. 2020,11(3):288–95. https://doi.org/10.1136/bmjspcare-2020-002333. Epub ahead of print.
9. Committee on Hospital Care. American Academy of Pediatrics. Family-centered care and the pediatrician's role. Pediatrics. 2003;112(3 Pt 1):691–7.
10. MacKenzie AR, Lasota M. Bringing life to death: the need for honest, compassionate, and effective end-of-life conversations. Am Soc Clin Oncol Educ Book. 2020;40:1–9. https://doi.org/10.1200/EDBK_279767.

11. Sutherland R. Dying well-informed: the need for better clinical education surrounding facilitating end-of-life conversations. Yale J Biol Med. 2019;92(4):757–64.
12. Weissman DE, Derse A. Informed consent in palliative care: part II #165. J Palliat Med. 2011;14(9):1066–7. https://doi.org/10.1089/jpm.2011.9651.
13. Kemper BJ. Therapeutic listening: developing the concept. J Psychosoc Nurs Ment Health Serv. 1992;30(7):21–3.
14. Hauer JM, Wolfe J. Supportive and palliative care of children with metabolic and neurological diseases. Curr Opin Support Palliat Care. 2014;8(3):296–302. https://doi.org/10.1097/SPC.0000000000000063.
15. Kacperek L. Non-verbal communication: the importance of listening. Br J Nurs. 1997;6(5):275–9. https://doi.org/10.12968/bjon.1997.6.5.275.
16. Bellieni CV, Coradeschi C, Curcio MR, Grande E, Buonocore G. Consents or waivers of responsibility? Parents' information in NICU. Minerva Pediatr. 2018. https://doi.org/10.23736/S0026-4946.18.05084-3. Epub ahead of print.
17. Habiba MA. Examining consent within the patient-doctor relationship. J Med Ethics. 2000;26(3):183–7.
18. Katz J. Informed consent—must it remain a fairy tale? J Contemp Health Law Policy. 1994;10:69–91.

Managing Grief and Its Phases

5.1 The Phases of Grief

Throughout palliative care process, a "stone-guest" looms: mourning. It is the mourning of the parents, who elaborate the loss of the child; and the mourning of the children who will have to work out the loss of their health.

Grief is the psychological process that occurs after a terrible news or an event that implies an affective loss or abandonment. It is different for each person. It can give different emotional and physical symptoms such as anxiety, fear, guilt, confusion, denial, depression, sadness, and emotional shock.

The pain of a loss can be experienced not only after a death, but every time in life we have an experience of definitive interruption of something we were emotionally very attached to. It bewilders, it imposes to react or to adapt to a new situation, but this is not always simple: a beloved one does not exist anymore. It is a wound and, therefore, requires time to heal.

The grieving process has been thoroughly analyzed [1, 2], and this analysis showed that it is not a unique event, but it is composed of several phases, usually appearing in a precise sequence, though some exceptions can emerge [3] (Table 5.1, Fig. 5.1).

5.2 The Pathological Grief

Grief becomes pathological when, after a while, the person continues having the same depressive symptoms [4]. A loss not properly worked out often leads to emotional problems and even psychopathological disorders, after months or even years. However, a properly crafted grief improves future abilities to cope with situations of loss, frustration, or suffering. The expression at a social, familiar, and personal level of the emotions accompanying the feelings of loss, and the rituals that help to

© The Author(s), under exclusive license to Springer Nature Switzerland AG 2022
C. V. Bellieni, *A New Holistic-Evolutive Approach to Pediatric Palliative Care*, https://doi.org/10.1007/978-3-030-96256-2_5

Table 5.1 Phases or stages of grief

Denial: Disbelief is the first reaction to a blow from life. Denial is an unavoidable stepping stone that parents and children go through and from which they finally have to step out to digest the loss. What is denying? Denying is a way of telling reality to wait that we are not yet ready. The impact of the news is so strong that we stop listening, understanding, and thinking. It may happen that at first the blockage is so great that we cannot even feel it. Denial has the sense of giving us a truce. There are those who deny the loss but there are also those who, hastily accepting the harshness of reality, what they really try is to deny the pain.
Anger: Anger simply has to be recognized and accepted in order to get it out. It should not be feared or worse, condemned. All the anger that remains inside, that we try to deny or hide will crush us. Anger has a reason for being. It is asking for help. Anger means asking for help. It prompts us to react, gather strength, produce adrenaline to take other paths; when we are at the bottom of the hole it makes us gain momentum to float up. It is a weapon for survival.
Negotiation: It is the moment in which we fantasize about the idea of reversing the situation, it is possible to reach an agreement with whoever is necessary, even promising God what is necessary. Ways are sought to make the inevitable not possible. But this stage is short: thinking all day about solutions is really exhausting.
Fear or depression: People feel sadness, uncertainty about the future, emptiness, and deep pain. They feel exhausted and any task becomes complicated. "Life is crazy," "I will never be happy," "I will not find anyone the same" or "he will never return" is what is often repeated when the person is facing pain. But despite the fact that one may think that this will never end and that it will last forever, the reality is that only from this point we rebuild ourselves.
Acceptance: It is the last step of grief. It is never easy to accept that what was lost was lost, and there is no going back. We have the alternative of not accepting, but once we arrive here, we realize that if we do not do so, the price to pay is very high. Getting to this point requires a lot of work. It is with acceptance that the stones that we find in life can become also part of the path. The alternative is to continue hurting ourselves. Because depression and anxiety are ways in which one hurts oneself. Feeling that pain srikes everyone, is a way to put the grief back to its place, and to stop punishing oneself.

elaborate the process of adaptation to loss can prevent the development of pathological grief, and facilitate the natural grief process [5].

The duration of the grief is variable [6], it can last for months and even years. Most people elaborate their grief in an adequate way, but others do not achieve it; it is important, thus, to know and spot the symptoms of anxiety and depression. When these symptoms end up taking over the person with a strong feeling of guilt and self-reproach and they rest constant, they highlight a pathological state.

One of the most important symptoms is improper anger. Anger can sometimes become a desire for revenge, prompting the person to carry it out against someone, often innocent. Some examples: traumatic marital breakups after the loss of a child; persecution and harassment of the doctor, sometimes leading to denouncing them unjustly. Displaying anger improperly will force the patient to remain indefinitely on one step of the grief elaboration, it will prevent them from turning the page and moving on with their lives [7]. In fact, what distinguishes normal from pathological

5.2 The Pathological Grief

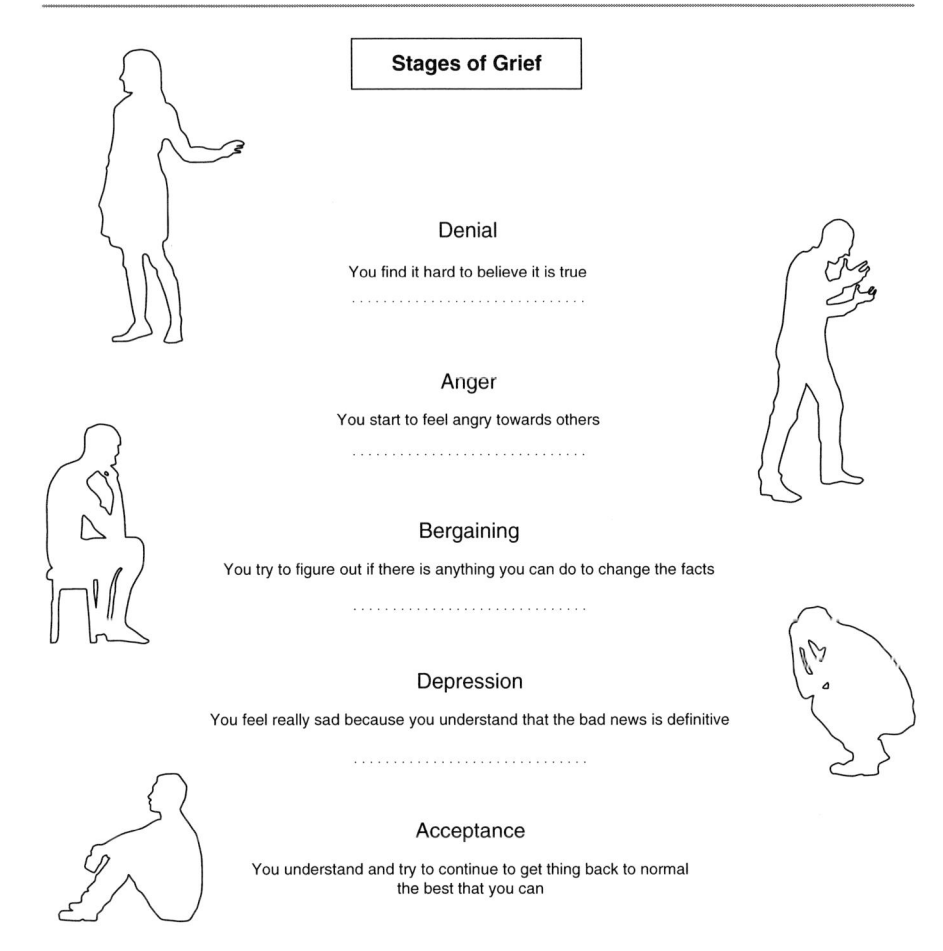

Stages of Grief

Denial
You find it hard to believe it is true

Anger
You start to feel angry towards others

Bergaining
You try to figure out if there is anything you can do to change the facts

Depression
You feel really sad because you understand that the bad news is definitive

Acceptance
You understand and try to continue to get thing back to normal the best that you can

Fig. 5.1 The phases of grief

grief is that the person remains stuck in one of the aforementioned steps (phases): the internal elaborations, instead of producing changes to advance to the next phases, paralyze the course of the normal grief.

Western societies do not help a good evolution of grief. These "societies of forced happiness" [8] do not allow people to be sad. Grief is unglamorous and showing fragility is considered impolite, because everyone fear that someone else's pain could awaken theirs. Those affected by the grief are therefore inundated with messages such as "come on, it's not that bad," "That happened a long time ago,, "Look at the bright side," and a great amount of energy is invested to deny and censure grief. But a censored grief will reappear often under other appearances, sometimes under the form of psychosomatic symptoms of nevroses [9].

Complicated grief is a recently recognized condition that occurs in about 7% of bereaved people [10]. People with this condition are caught up in rumination about the circumstances of the death, worry about its consequences, or excessive avoidance of reminders of the loss. Unable to acknowledge the actual features of their loss, they, need help, and clinicians need to know how to recognize the symptoms and how to provide help [11].

5.3 Communicating with the Depressed Child or Parent

The major depressive disorder is a common and serious medical illness that negatively affects how you feel, the way you think and how you act. Fortunately, it is also treatable. Depression causes feelings of sadness and/or a loss of interest in activities you once enjoyed [12, 13]. The death of a loved one, the loss of a job, or the ending of a relationship are difficult experiences for a person to endure. It is normal for feelings of sadness or grief to develop in response to such situations. Those experiencing loss often might describe themselves as being "depressed." But being sad is not the same as having depression. The grieving process is natural and unique to each individual and shares some features of depression. Both grief and depression may involve intense sadness and withdrawal from usual activities, but they are different under important aspects [13]:

- In grief, painful feelings come in waves, often intermixed with positive memories of the deceased. In major depression, mood and/or interest (pleasure) are decreased for most of the time.
- In grief, self-esteem is usually maintained. In major depression, feelings of worthlessness and self-loathing are common.
- In grief, thoughts of death may surface in order to "joining" the deceased loved one. In major depression, thoughts are focused on ending one's life due to feeling worthless or undeserving of living or being unable to cope with the pain of depression.

Grief and depression can co-exist. For some people, the pain of the death of a loved one, of losing a job or being a victim of a physical assault or a major disaster can lead to depression. When grief and depression co-occur, the grief is more severe and lasts longer than grief without depression. Distinguishing between grief and depression is important and can assist people in getting the help, the support or treatment they need [12].

5.4 The Experience of Loss

In his Man's Search for Meaning [14], Victor Frankl argued that people are driven by a deep and inescapable need to find or create a sense of meaning and purpose in their life, and this drive can facilitate their ability to cope with and even transcend the most horrible experiences. This theme has struck a deep chord not only in psychology, and has been applied to numerous experiences of human suffering, including the experience of mourning. As a result, research in the field of bereavement and loss has begun to examine the ways in which mourners seek meaning in the aftermath of the loss of loved ones [15]. An attentive clinical psychiatrist, aware of this, can intervene by facilitating the reconstruction of new meanings in critical moments and in the most appropriate ways. For example, evidence provided by Davis and colleagues [16, 17] suggests that making sense of loss is associated with less distress in the first year after loss. Thus, a psychiatrist can effectively intervene by listening to and exploring the sense of purpose the patient glimpses, begins to intuit, or brings back to consciousness from his or her past [18]. To this end, the clinician might encourage the survivor to continue his or her dialog with the deceased, in the form of letters or inner speech or prayer or meditation. Several narrative exercises have been developed [18] that can be used as self-help strategies in bereavement or in the context of bereavement therapy. The potential value of such methods is suggested by a recent randomized controlled study conducted by Shear and his colleagues [11] which demonstrates the efficacy of the evocative telling of the death story and promotes a connection with the deceased (e.g., through the use of imaginary conversations) and the reformulation of life goals.

However, the road is long. Before reaching recovery and control, the sense of loss leads to "self-death" [19] or "self-loss" [20]: the "self" is lost, and the lost self is replaced by a void, sometimes by a ghost, and from a deep sense of sadness, of loss of meaning, which can lead to despair, making the person extremely vulnerable to the outside world. The survivor, but also those who suffer a loss due to their own illness, feel a sense of deep anguish and a sense of unbridgeable emptiness, of emotional drying up and disinterest in everything that surrounds them. The self is now dominated by a sense of helplessness.

There is a weakening of the volitional capacity, or *abulia* [21], which makes the person feel a sense of helplessness and loss of vital energy, a reduced interest and a reduced ability to carry out the usual daily activities. Thoughts flow with increasing difficulty, disrupting questions of self-accusation up to the conviction of deserving extreme punishment and the search for death as a way of expiation.

The sense of guilt thus overlaps with impotence. The inability to control one's mood and to help oneself leads the person to express a negative judgment about themselves, which is expressed through fear for the future, frustration, and anger towards themselves and others. Loneliness, anger and a sense of helplessness are the key words in this phase.

The above allows us to understand how difficult and often frustrating it can be to establish a helping relationship with a person who is experiencing a depressive experience, a person who suffers deeply, locked up in a world from which they cannot communicate, that isolates them from others, from which they feel neither understood nor accepted. Often, albeit different in intensities, the person who is going through the depressive experience enters a negative spiral characterized by resistance to any attempt to help, which induces in those who offer help, a reaction of rejection and intolerance, leading to accuse the suffering person. Another frequent reaction of those who offer help is the overstimulation of the depressed, through continuous stimuli, mostly superficial or provocative, which reinforce the sense of guilt and inadequacy felt by the person, creating a vicious circle.

The support of the depressed parent or child by the staff of the pediatric palliative care is fundamental. Caregivers must base the therapeutic relationship on the acceptance of the depressed person in his immobility and in his impossibility of planning a future, aware that this is due to the psychopathological condition, and that the person is not guilty of it. Although appearing refractory to relational stress, the depressed person is very receptive to any manifestation of attention; for this reason it is necessary to guarantee them a sincere and available presence.

5.5 The Risk of Suicide

One of the risks not to be underestimated, especially in the most severe depressive episodes, is suicide, used as a maladaptive coping strategy that occurs in the presence of excessively low levels of self-esteem [22]. Suicide is a way to permanently cancel the feelings of inadequacy and guilt. The greatest risk does not manifest itself only in the extreme phase of depression, during which the person does not have the necessary strength to program or implement the suicidal intention, but also in the first moments of improvement, in which they begin to recover energy which can be used to realize self-suppressive intentions [23]. People who report feeling lonely after a sudden bereavement are more likely to attempt suicide, and in this, the size and quality of their acquaintance network is important [24]. People with personality disorders are more prone to suicide after bereavement [25]. It is necessary not to underestimate this risk and to resort to the intervention of the specialist as soon as the first signs are perceived.

5.6 Interventions Aimed at the Family

The interventions aimed at the family are essentially informative-educational on the evolution of the depressive problem, and on the possible support aimed at involving them in the treatment project. The person going through the depressive experience hanges his/her role within the family, with important repercussions on the functioning of the family unit, which in turn is forced to restructure, perhaps only temporarily, the roles within it [26]. The family must be considered an important resource to be involved in the health recovery process [27].

5.7 Interventions Aimed at Caregivers

Assisting a person while going through a depressive experience is a difficult and emotionally engaging experience, which can produce feelings of aggression, rejection, and frustration. The treating staff must therefore have tools to become aware of the experiences that the relationship with the depressed person induces in them, and at the same time to use these experiences for the sake of the patient [28]. In addition to independently seeking a balance and confronting with the out-of-hospital reality, the comparison and discussion within the care staff are useful tools of help. Other more structured tools are support groups and supervision [29]. The use of these support tools involves discussing in a group that affects the most personal sphere of the professional, such as the emotions that the difficult relationships arouse.

References

1. Buglass E. Grief and bereavement theories. Nurs Stand. 2010;24(41):44–7. https://doi.org/10.7748/ns2010.06.24.41.44.c7834.
2. Corr CA. Elisabeth Kübler-Ross and the "Five Stages" Model in a Sampling of Recent American Textbooks. Omega (Westport). 2020;82(2):294–322. https://doi.org/10.1177/0030222818809766. Epub 2018 Nov 15.
3. Kubler-Ross E. On death and dying. Scribner Ed; 1969.
4. Zisook S, DeVaul R. Unresolved grief. Am J Psychoanal. 1985;45(4):370–9.
5. Horowitz MJ, Bonanno GA, Holen A. Pathological grief: diagnosis and explanation. Psychosom Med. 1993;55(3):260–73. https://doi.org/10.1097/00006842-199305000-00004.
6. Bryant RA. Is pathological grief lasting more than 12 months grief or depression? Curr Opin Psychiatry. 2013;26(1):41–6. https://doi.org/10.1097/YCO.0b013e32835b2ca2.
7. Comtesse H, Vogel A, Kersting A, Rief W, Steil R, Rosner R. When does grief become pathological? Evaluation of the ICD-11 diagnostic proposal for prolonged grief in a treatment-seeking sample. Eur J Psychotraumatol. 2020;11(1):1694348. https://doi.org/10.1080/20008198.2019.1694348.
8. Khodus HV. FORCED HAPPINESS AS A MODERN SOCIO AND CULTURAL IMPERATIVE. Anthropol Meas Philos Res. 2015;8:64–73.
9. Zisook S, Simon NM, Reynolds CF 3rd, Pies R, Lebowitz B, Young IT, Madowitz J, Shear MK. Bereavement, complicated grief, and DSM, part 2: complicated grief. J Clin Psychiatry. 2010;71(8):1097–8. https://doi.org/10.4088/JCP.10ac06391blu.
10. Kersting A, Brähler E, Glaesmer H, Wagner B. Prevalence of complicated grief in a representative population-based sample. J Affect Disord. 2011;131(1–3):339–43. https://doi.org/10.1016/j.jad.2010.11.032. Epub 2011 Jan 8.
11. Shear K, Frank E, Houck PR, Reynolds CF. Treatment of complicated grief: a randomized controlled trial. J Am Med Assoc. 2005;293:2601–8.
12. American Psychiatric Association. Diagnostic and statistical manual of mental disorders (DSM-5). 5th ed; 2013.
13. American Psychiatric Association. What is Depression? 2021. https://www.psychiatry.org/patients-families/depression/what-is-depression
14. Frankl V. Man's search for meaning. New York: Touchstone Books; 1962.
15. Gillies J, Neimeyer RA. Loss, grief, and the search for significance: toward a model of meaning reconstruction in bereavement. J Constr Psychol. 2006;19(1):31–65.
16. Davis CG, Nolen-Hoeksema S. Loss and meaning: how do people make sense of loss? Am Behav Sci. 2001;44:726–41.
17. Davis CG, Nolen-Hoeksema S, Larson J. Making sense of loss and benefiting from the experience: two construals of meaning. J Pers Soc Psychol. 1998;75:561–74.
18. Neimeyer RA. Searching for the meaning of meaning: grief therapy and the process of reconstruction. Death Stud. 2000;24:541–58.
19. Beck CT. Teetering on the edge: a substantive theory of postpartum depression. Nurs Res. 1993;42:42–8.
20. Chernomas WM. Experiencing depression: women's perspectives in recovery. J Psychiatr Ment Health Nurs. 1997;4(6):393–400.
21. Stroebe M, Boelen PA, van den Hout M, Stroebe W, Salemink E, van den Bout J. Ruminative coping as avoidance. A reinterpretation of its function in adjustment to bereavement. Eur Arch Psychiatry Clin Neurosci. 2007;257:462–72.

22. Bhullar N, Sanford RL, Maple M. Profiling suicide exposure risk factors for psychological distress: an empirical test of the proposed continuum of survivorship model. Front Psych. 2021;12:692363. https://doi.org/10.3389/fpsyt.2021.692363.
23. Takahashi J. Depression and suicide. JMAJ. 2001;44(8):359–63.
24. Pitman AL, King MB, Marston L, Osborn DPJ. The association of loneliness after sudden bereavement with risk of suicide attempt: a nationwide survey of bereaved adults. Soc Psychiatry Psychiatr Epidemiol. 2020;55(8):1081–92. https://doi.org/10.1007/s00127-020-01921-w. Epub 2020 Jul 18.
25. Zabihi S, Jones R, Moran P, King M, Osborn D, Pitman A. The association between personality disorder traits and suicidality following sudden bereavement: a national cross-sectional survey. J Personal Disord. 2021:1–19. https://doi.org/10.1521/pedi_2021_35_520. Epub ahead of print.
26. Reiss-Brennan B, Oppenheim D, Kirstein JL. Rebuilding family relationship competencies as a primary health intervention. Prim Care Companion J Clin Psychiatry. 2002;4(2):41–53. https://doi.org/10.4088/pcc.v04n0202.
27. Smith-MacDonald L, Venturato L, Hunter P, Kaasalainen S, Sussman T, McCleary L, Thompson G, Wickson-Griffiths A, Sinclair S. Perspectives and experiences of compassion in long-term care facilities within Canada: a qualitative study of patients, family members and health care providers. BMC Geriatr. 2019;19(1):128. https://doi.org/10.1186/s12877-019-1135-x.
28. Menthies LI. Staff support systems: task and antitask in adolescent institutions. In: Containing anxiety in institutions. London: Free Associations Books; 1989.
29. Simpson-Southward C, Waller G, Hardy GE. Supervision for treatment of depression: an experimental study of the role of therapist gender and anxiety. Behav Res Ther. 2016;77:17–22.

Challenges in Communication with Parents and Children

6.1 It Is Difficult to Use the Word Death…

Talking about death is usually devastating, so much so that, in Western society, death tends to be exorcized. Little is said about it: horror films multiply, to "get vaccinated" against shocking events; metaphors and synonyms are used to indicate death, such as "they have disappeared," "they have passed away," not to mention the unpronounceable word "tumor" [1]; but it remains a taboo. Death is a ghost, a taboo, something mysterious, hidden, very well hidden; so, when it arrives, it is scary and crushing [2]. In Western society, death is simply not foreseen, it is not allowed, it is not accepted [3]. In the past, grandparents were commonly seen dying at home, the wake was participated by the whole family, and the dying often passed by in awareness. Today, the death process is completely hospitalized, aseptic, medicalized, relegated to loneliness, and the ideal is not to die with the loved ones, but to die without realizing it, all of a sudden, or anesthetized [4]. When death is communicated, one must know that it is a forbidden word, an insult, a curse, a rudeness.

So, when we start talking about a baby's death, we should realize that we are using the most natural and at the same time most alien word possible. We are starting a speech in a foreign language for those who are listening. Hence, this term should be introduced gradually, with circumspection and great caution. Therefore, many caregivers experience a heavy burden during the end-of-life process, and the unpronounceable word "death" is the first difficult step to overcome. Many healthcare professionals feel themselves unprepared to communicate to patients and families the complex issues of death and dying. They attribute it to the fact that these topics were not discussed or only briefly discussed during formal university education [5]. Now is the time to destroy a myth: death is a characteristic of the human presence on earth; death is the end that comes sooner or later. It is physiological, natural, and good for the next generations [6]. It is also an event full of pain, suffering, and regret; but it is normal, this is how difficult situations can find an end and

---

© The Author(s), under exclusive license to Springer Nature Switzerland AG 2022
C. V. Bellieni, *A New Holistic-Evolutive Approach to Pediatric Palliative Care*, https://doi.org/10.1007/978-3-030-96256-2_6

the new generations can find their place. It is not to be rushed or sought; it is an inevitable drama that must be learned, recognized, and accepted, as thousands of millions of people have done so far.

6.2   ... Much More That of a Child

If death is a forbidden word in Western culture [7], the association of death with the idea of a child is absolutely unthinkable. Everything has assured you that you will live in a medically perfect world, where death and disease are all under control, and suddenly the death of a child makes this perfect building collapse. You do not only refuse it: you cannot even imagine it [8]. For this reason, the field of pediatric palliative care is a minefield: it dares what cannot be dared, it talks about what should not be talked about. Once there were sexual taboos; today, the taboo is the idea of perfection and invulnerability that society has created, and the idea of the child as a product. In this, the numerous prenatal, and postnatal examinations, support a false reassurance on the child's future. Maybe because any parent sees and listens only to what they want to see and hear. The child has become a kind of product, in Western societies; it is the "icing on the cake" one puts over after having established one's career; they are usually unique, and born when the parents are over 30, in Europe. So it is expected that, if this is the norm, if everyone do so, babies also have a guarantee of perfection, a sort of certificate of invulnerability. The child's illness collapses this dogma.

Imagine then how unthinkable it is to speak of illness and death to a child. We will see later on in this book how to do it. The way of sharing information with children about their disease and prognosis has changed substantially over the past 70 years. Until the 1960s, the prevalent practice was to hide the diagnosis to the minor, or to hide its life-threatening nature, to protect children from fear. In the decades since, the importance of children's awareness has been increasingly recognized, in part as a reflection of the advances in medical care (and of improved children survival) and in part for a better awareness of how children understand diseases and death [9]. The debate has evolved into a more nuanced and personalized consideration of what, when and how much a child should be told about their diagnosis [10]; however, it is not surprising that parents often try to protect their children from what they think is emotionally overwhelming [11]. The current trend is to avoid simple "on-off" recommendations.

Studies show that talking about death with a child shouldn't be a taboo for parents; no parent has regretted dealing with this with their dying child [12]; however, it is not yet clear how disrupting is the impact for the child of receiving bad news.

The guidelines of the National Institute for Excellence in Health and Care (NICE) recommend that in the case of children with life-limiting diseases, the information should take into account both their age and their level of understanding [13], and of their cognitive, emotional, and psychological development [14] as we will see below.

6.3 Should We Talk of Their Death and Disease?

It is important to consider what to say to the child. This is an old problem: should we say the truth to the child? Two points matter in dealing with this topic.

The first is considering three aspects of the matter: (a) what they understand; (b) if becoming aware of bad news will improve their state; (c) our duty of being always honest with the children. Point (a) seems obvious: if a baby does not understand at all what we will be saying, speaking is useless; but throughout their development, children change, they vary their attitudes and skills, and our approach should change. Point (b) is crucial: is it useful for a baby who does not understand what death is, to know they are going to die? Point (c): If the information can be counterproductive, it can utterly be avoided without infringing the moral duty of honesty.

The second point worth considering is that what matters and makes the difference is not always what we say, but how we are perceived. Kenneth Nunn, in a recent paper on this matter, wrote that "Interaction is more important than information" [15]. In fact, the most important point in bad-news communication to a child is not the accuracy in giving data or figures, but what they perceive from our behavior. In other words, some teenagers can be longing for a thorough description of what they are going through, others don't; the rate of younger children who want to receive accurate information is lower than adolescents, but some can have benefit from it; however, all want to perceive care and not abandon, closeness and respect of their intimacy, in the form due to their mood, age, and character.

Anyway, little is known about the kids' point of view about receiving bad news on their health; widespread reluctance to conduct research on this issue and in particular on children with terminal illnesses, has hampered further study. Thus, we should rely on what we know from the studies performed on parents, and from the few ones performed on children.

From the parents' point of view, the answer is yes: it is better for parents that their children know the truth. Speaking of death with their children will help parents to blunt the loss [16]. One study examined this, through the experiences of the parents of children who died of cancer. Kreicbergs et al. surveyed the parents of Swedish children who had died of terminal cancer between 1992 and 1997, and found that those who discussed their child's imminent death had a much less complicated bereavement process and less regret than those who did not (2004). More specifically, 27% of those who did not talk about death with their child regretted that choice. Parents who sense that their child is aware of his or her imminent death, more often later regret not having talked with their child than do parents who could talk of this with their child; overall, in this study no parent regretted having talked with his or her child about death [12].

The limited research on children's preferences on this matter indicates that in most cases they prefer to know. Clinicians generally agree that children should be informed about their prognosis and will benefit from open communication about their impending death [17, 18]. However, it is hard to assess the benefit a child can get from becoming aware of their imminent death. As a rule of thumb, a recommendation can be given: to "disclose the evidence when the evidence has become evident," i.e., when the child has evident suspects on their possible bad prognosis or their imminent death. Anyway, parents may hesitate about if, when, and how to broach bad news with dying children [16]. By the late 1980s, the recommended approach to prognostic disclosure in pediatrics fluctuated from "never tell" to "always tell"; in recent years, however, there has been a growing appreciation for the sincere disclosure of bad news in pediatrics [10]. Anyway, it is important to avoid the suspect that you are lying to them; mistrust and all the possible consequences this may have, complicate the relationships and exacerbate the stress, the suffering, and the discomfort of the child.

Last, communication models rarely consider the potential influence of children's previous experiences and exposure to illness and death on their understanding of these concepts. Empirical studies indicate that children who have had a previous experience of death (those who live in areas where disease or armed conflicts are endemic) have a relatively advanced understanding of death [9], and this in some cases can help in communication, but not always: it depends on how these previous experiences have been felt and remembered.

6.4   Speaking According to the Patient's Character

Doctors rarely try to know the character of the person they are dealing with, though speaking according to the character of the patient is useful in order not to fall into incommunicability. Some references are useful to identify the patient's character, to address them appropriately. This approach is useful when you talk either with the parents or with children.

Different types of personalities exist, described by the philosopher Gustaf Jung [19] and later elaborated by the Myers-Briggs couple in the past century. The Myers-Briggs Type Indicator or, more briefly, the Myers-Briggs Indicator, is a personality test designed to help identify some of the most important personal preferences of the patient [20, 21]. The Indicator was created by Katharine Cook Briggs and her daughter Isabel Briggs Myers during World War II. We can so summarize their work, by saying that two main characters exist: extroverts and introverts. Then there are four subtypes: we have the synthetic, the analytical, the suspicious, and the trusting character. These authors described these types carefully and their final approach is reported in Table 6.1. We should use these parameters for a tailored approach, not to adapt forcefully our way of speaking; the aim of these references is not to simulate acquaintance, but to respect the patient's way of interacting, to intercept their hidden vocabulary made of silences, grimaces, and cries. If we can manage this, then a shy patient will not be hit aggressively with multiple redundant news, and an aggressive one will not be informed with half words, or defensively. An analytical person will ask for a lot of data, a synthetic person only asks for a clear and concise picture of the situation, and these features should be promptly acknowledged and satisfied (Table 6.1).

6.5 Obstacles to Communication

Table 6.1 Meyers-Briggs personality types. In the table on the right, under any "type" its main features are reported. In the column on the left, further descriptions of the "types" appear

Outwardly or Inwardly focused : Extroversion/Introversion	Extroversion	Introversion
	Initiating Active Enthusiastic Gregarious	Received Contained Intimate Reserved
Longing or not for explicit information : Sensing/Intuition	Sensing	Intuition
	Concrete Realistic Practical Traditional	Abstract Imaginative Conceptual Original
Eager or not in taking decisions : Thinking/Feeling	Thinking	Feeling
	Logical Reasonable Questioning Critical Tough	Empathetic Compassionate Empathetic Accepting Tender
Flexible or inflexible : Perceiving/Judging	Perceiving	Judging
	Casual Open-ended Pressure-prompted Spontaneous Emergent	Systematic Planning Early starting Scheduled Methodical

6.5 Obstacles to Communication

It is really difficult to talk to the child and their parents about the child's health bad news. Social and cultural reasons can be further obstacles, and it is necessary to know which they are.

1. *Cultural factors*

    Culture and traditions, ethnicity, religious, and spiritual beliefs will influence the perspectives of children and parents or caregivers about the meaning of death and illness (e.g., there is a possible reluctance in some religious communities to reveal a terminal condition because it could exclude hope and faith). Conceptual interpretations of death vary widely throughout the world; for example, in South Africa a study described how death can be seen as a transformative experience [22]. This requires to explore an individual's belief system, and at the same time to ensure stereotypes on any religious belief to be avoided.

2. *Children's factors*

    Although several children and adolescents desire information about their disease (including whether or not they may die), this is not universal. In one of the few studies that address this issue, 100 survivors of childhood cancer between the ages of 11 and 20 years were surveyed on various aspects of end-of-life care. Ninety-six percent thought that a child has a right to know if he or she is terminally ill. When asked if they would want to know if they were terminally ill, 85% said they would, 12% replied no, and 2.5% were not sure [23]. Some childhood cancer survivors reported that their limited knowledge of their illness at the time helped them cope with it [24].

A retrospective study of 86 bereaved parents [9] found that those ($n = 55$) who did not speak to their children about death had based their decision on the perception that their child did not want to talk about his/her own death. Children may be unwilling to speak up or feel inhibited in raising concerns, especially if they are aware of adults' anxiety and discomfort around the topic [25].

3. *Education of parents or caregivers and sociodemographic history*

   The educational level of the parents or caregivers can affect the communication although the literature is inconsistent on this.

   A cross-sectional study of caregiver-child HIV-positive dyads in Ethiopia found higher disclosure rates among illiterate caregivers than among caregivers with a higher level of education, and most parents preferred to disclose the news of the bad prognosis when their child was older than 14 years [26]. A similar result was observed in a Thai study [27] on 103 caregivers of HIV-infected children (aged 6–16 years). In contrast, a study in the United States found that children who knew their HIV status were more likely to come from families with a higher socioeconomic status [28].

4. *Desire to protect the child from distress.*

   Parents or guardians may not appreciate the potential importance of communication and often express a desire of protecting their child, fearing that the disclosure would have negative psychological consequences for their child, such as distress, depression, anxiety, isolation, and loss of hope. Other parents report that they did not want to challenge their own or their children's hopes that the disease could be cured [29]. In conclusion, for some parents, death is not considered an appropriate topic to discuss with children.

   Parents or caregivers of children with HIV sometimes fear that the disclosure would induce children to ask difficult questions about the source of HIV and would blame, resent, or lose respect for their parents. The stigma associated with HIV-positive status may raise concerns in parents or caregivers that the child would disclose their status to others, with negative consequences not only for the child but for the entire family [30]. Similar feelings have not been reported in the cancer literature.

5. *Parents' emotional well-being*

   Parents' mental health could also affect communication. A cross-sectional study in the United States on 94 children (5–18 years) with cancer and their mothers [31] found that mothers' symptoms of depression were associated with their communication style (e.g., disinterest in discussion of the disease with the children). Observers rated mothers with more symptoms of depression as having a more negative communication style and being less friendly, understanding and receptive when interacting with their baby.

6. *Health professionals*
The contribution of health professionals to the triad that participates in communication (child, parent, and health worker) is also influenced by their own beliefs, their cultural and religious context, their experience and knowledge, both in professional and personal sense [29]. Obstacles by health professionals also include a lack of training for discussions and a reluctance to face a family's "avoidant communication model"; unrealistic parental expectations, clinical uncertainty, and a lack of cultural support impair this reluctance.

There are specific stressors which can affect the ability of a healthcare professional to communicate effectively with their patients [32]. These include: frequent exposure to death, lack of time to devote to dying patients, increased workload, initial symptoms of burnout, but also the utopian desire to "continue as usual" [33] after giving the bad news. Frequent exposure to death could trigger memories of unresolved losses to the healthcare worker [34]. Healthcare professionals may feel helpless because they have not been able to prevent the death of a child or avoid emotional distress to the family. The emotional effect of these problems can make healthcare workers feel inadequate to support the children, their parents or other healthcare workers, and could contribute to high levels of psychological morbidity, as was reported among doctors and among medical university students [35]. Some strategies that healthcare professionals can adopt to manage their feelings of grief in response to these difficult situations can lead to creating a physical or emotional distance between them and the family through impatience or formality, which can make communication even more difficult. But there are also positive and useful strategies, that we will describe later in this book.

However, there is evidence that healthcare professionals involved in palliative care have similar or slightly lower levels of stress and burnout than their peers in other specialties [36] and half than of those working in intensive care units [37]. This finding could show that factors within the palliative care service, such as high-quality support from staff, mitigate some of the stressors associated with working with dying patients. These observations indicate that psychological support is critical for healthcare professionals facing life-threatening conditions.

6.6 What Helps in Communicating Bad News on Their Health to the Children?

The terrible news of a bad prognosis can find one defense: a well-structured ego. And for a well-structured ego, a well-structured family is needed, and a childhood that made children know their own importance, that they are desired without being owned. It is crucial for the child having felt that they can be wanted and desired without being possessed [38]. This happens if the family has done a work of osmotic education: showing unity without eager possession, love without senses of guilt. I have written "osmotic education," because the true educator is not who speaks, but who shows what and how to do; the best education is inducing imitation rather than obedience. This is why, the emotional history of the family, child's previous experiences and traumas, what parents communicated to the children in their first few years, should be investigated to predict the reactions to grief.

Emotional hygiene must be cultivated in all families. The feeling of being wanted is an elixir for the child; the feeling of being owned, of being a project is deleterious. For the child, how life of their earliest years was spent is fundamental.

The concept that someone might disappear, the acceptance of detachment and departure is built throughout the first few years of life. Playing hide and seek with their parents, [39], or letting the objects they threw disappear and reappear, (in order to learn that they themselves can disappear and reappear) is a training for future losses. If children have received the certainty of being able to disappear without leaving trauma, the trauma of change and isolation in hospital will be less hard to accept. Trust is built in the first few years of life and its trace is indelible, in good or in bad sense. A trustful spirit makes the difference; of course, even such confident individuals can get deep wounds by a sudden news of a terminal illness, but they are usually stronger than those who have a frail personality.

If, on the other hand, parents have stuck in their children a sense of panic in the early stages of life, due to their absence or their omnipresence, any loss will be a trauma [40].

A well-structured ego is necessary for health professionals as well, even in order to giving bad news. How many doctors receive an affective care during their career to be capable of this?

6.7 Special Children

The specific needs of children with cognitive or sensory disabilities must also be taken into account, when dialoguing with them. In the case of children with mental diseases, the possibility of communicating with them should not be ruled out. Obviously, this will happen in a special way, without the aim of explaining difficult things or - sometimes - of obtaining a conscient consent. Every contact and every communication should be respectful and should avoid in them the idea of being mocked or neglected. Cancer professionals should assess the special information needs of people with an intellectual disability [41].

Children with sensory disabilities are another special group in the range of communicative problems. Their communication needs are often not met in healthcare settings, and this could negatively affect their outcomes. Thus, every effort should be done to find the correct way of appropriately communicating with them.

References

1. Hershenov DB. The death of a person. J Med Philos. 2006;31(2):107–20.
2. Markin RD, Zilcha-Mano S. Cultural processes in psychotherapy for perinatal loss: breaking the cultural taboo against perinatal grief. Psychotherapy (Chic). 2018;55(1):20–6. https://doi.org/10.1037/pst0000122.
3. Allan K. Forbidden words: taboo and the censoring of language. Cambridge University Press; 2006.
4. Testoni I, Cordioli C, Nodari E, Zsak E, Marinoni G, Venturini D, Maccarini A. Language re-discovered: a death education intervention in the net between Kindergarten, Family and Territory. Ital J Sociol Educ. 2019;11:331–46.
5. Oates JR, Maani CV. Death and dying. In: StatPearls [Internet]. Treasure Island, FL: StatPearls Publishing; 2020.
6. Fries J. Aging, natural death, and the compression of morbidity. N Engl J Med. 1980;303:130–5. https://doi.org/10.1056/NEJM198007173030304.
7. De Clercq E, Rost M, Rakic M, et al. The conceptual understanding of pediatric palliative care: a Swiss healthcare perspective. BMC Palliat Care. 2019;18:55.
8. Nuss SL. Redefining parenthood: surviving the death of a child. Cancer Nurs. 2014;37(1):E51–60. https://doi.org/10.1097/NCC.0b013e3182a0da1f.
9. Stein A, Dalton L, Rapa E, Bluebond-Langner M, Hanington L, Stein KF, Ziebland S, Rochat T, Harrop E, Kelly B, Bland R, Communication Expert Group. Communication with children and adolescents about the diagnosis of their own life threatening condition. Lancet. 2019;393(10176):1150–63. https://doi.org/10.1016/S0140-6736(18)33201-X. Epub 2019 Mar 14.
10. Sisk BA, Bluebond-Langner M, Wiener L, Mack J, Wolfe J. Prognostic disclosures to children: a historical perspective. Pediatrics. 2016;138(3):e20161278. https://doi.org/10.1542/peds.2016-1278. Epub 2016 Aug 25.
11. Rost M, Mihailov E. In the name of the family? Against parents' refusal to disclose prognostic information to children. Med Health Care Philos. 2021;24(3):421–32. https://doi.org/10.1007/s11019-021-10017-4.
12. Kreicbergs U, Valdimarsdottir U, Onelov E, Henter JI, Steineck G. Talking about death with children who have severe malignant disease. N Engl J Med. 2004;351(12):1175–86. https://doi.org/10.1056/NEJMoa040366.
13. NICE. End of life care for infants, children and young people with life-limiting conditions: planning and management. 2019. https://www.nice.org.uk/guidance/ng61
14. Coad J, Kaur J, Ashley N, Owens C, Hunt A, Chambers L, Brown E. Exploring the perceived met and unmet need of life-limited children, young people and families. J Pediatr Nurs. 2015;30(1):45–53. https://doi.org/10.1016/j.pedn.2014.09.007. Epub 2014 Sep 28.
15. Nunn K. Delivering bad news. J Paediatr Child Health. 2019;55(6):617–20.
16. Kushnick HL. Trusting them with the truth-disclosure and the good death for children with terminal illness. Virtual Mentor. 2010;12(7):573–7. https://doi.org/10.1001/virtualmentor.2010.12.7.msoc1-1007.
17. Hinds PS, Drew D, Oakes LL, et al. End-of-life preferences of pediatric patients with cancer. J Clin Oncol. 2005a;23(36):9153.
18. Hinds PS, Schum L, Baker JN, Wolfe J. Key factors affecting dying children and their families. J Palliat Med. 2005b;8(Suppl 1):S70–8. https://doi.org/10.1089/jpm.2005.8.s-70.
19. Jung CG. Psychological types. London: Routledge; 1999.
20. Myers IB, McCaulley MH, Quenk NL, Hammer AL. MBTI_Manual: a guide to the development and use of the Myers-Briggs type indicator. 3rd ed. Palo Alto, CA: Consulting Psychologists Press; 1998.

21. Myers IB, Myers PB. Gifts differing: understanding personality type. Palo Alto, CA: Consulting Psychologists Press; 1993.
22. Ekore RI, Lanre-Abass B. African Cultural Concept of Death and the Idea of Advance Care Directives. Indian J Palliat Care. 2016;22(4):369–72. https://doi.org/10.4103/0973-1075.191741.
23. de Vos MA, van der Heide A, Maurice-Stam H, et al. The process of end-of-life decision-making in pediatrics: a national survey in the Netherlands. Pediatrics. 2011;127:e1004–12.
24. Jacobs S, Perez J, Cheng YI, Sill A, Wang J, Lyon ME. Adolescent end of life preferences and congruence with their parents' preferences: results of a survey of adolescents with cancer. Pediatr Blood Cancer. 2015;62(4):710–4. https://doi.org/10.1002/pbc.25358. Epub 2014 Dec 24.
25. Aldridge J, Shimmon K, Miller M, Fraser LK, Wright B. 'I can't tell my child they are dying'. Helping parents have conversations with their child. Arch Dis Child Educ Pract Ed. 2017;102:182–7.
26. Biadgilign S, Deribew A, Amberbir A, Escudero HR, Deribe K. Factors associated with HIV/AIDS diagnostic disclosure to HIV infected children receiving HAART: a multi-center study in Addis Ababa, Ethiopia. PLoS One. 2011;6(3):e17572.
27. Oberdorfer P, Puthanakit T, Louthrenoo O, Charnsil C, Sirisanthana V, Sirisanthana T. Disclosure of HIV/AIDS diagnosis to HIV-infected children in Thailand. J Paediatr Child Health. 2006;42(5):283–8. https://doi.org/10.1111/j.1440-1754.2006.00855.x.
28. Wiener L, Mellins CA, Marhefka S, Battles HB. Disclosure of an HIV diagnosis to children: history, current research, and future directions. J Dev Behav Pediatr. 2007;28(2):155–66. https://doi.org/10.1097/01.DBP.0000267570.87564.cd.
29. Hrdlickova L, Polakova K, Loucka M. Important aspects influencing delivery of serious news in pediatric oncology: a scoping review. Children (Basel). 2021;8(2):166. https://doi.org/10.3390/children8020166.
30. Qiao S, Li X, Stanton B. Disclosure of parental HIV infection to children: a systematic review of global literature. AIDS Behav. 2013;17(1):369–89. https://doi.org/10.1007/s10461-011-0069-x.
31. Rodriguez EM, Dunn MJ, Zuckerman T, Hughart L, Vannatta K, Gerhardt CA, Saylor M, Schuele CM, Compas BE. Mother-child communication and maternal depressive symptoms in families of children with cancer: integrating macro and micro levels of analysis. J Pediatr Psychol. 2013;38(7):732–43. https://doi.org/10.1093/jpepsy/jst018. Epub 2013 Apr 24.
32. Norouzinia R, Aghabarari M, Shiri M, Karimi M, Samami E. Communication Barriers Perceived by Nurses and Patients. Glob J Health Sci. 2015;8(6):65–74. https://doi.org/10.5539/gjhs.v8n6p65.
33. Ha JF, Longnecker N. Doctor-patient communication: a review. Ochsner J. 2010;10(1):38–43.
34. Shanfield SB. The mourning of the health care professional: an important element in education about death and loss. Death Educ. 1981;4(4):385–95. https://doi.org/10.1080/07481188108253357.
35. Imo UO. Burnout and psychiatric morbidity among doctors in the UK: a systematic literature review of prevalence and associated factors. BJPsych Bull. 2017;41(4):197–204.
36. Berman R, Campbell M, Makin W, Todd C. Occupational stress in palliative medicine, medical oncology and clinical oncology specialist registrars. Clin Med (Lond). 2007;7(3):235–42. https://doi.org/10.7861/clinmedicine.7-3-235.
37. Martins Pereira S, Teixeira CM, Carvalho AS, Hernández-Marrero P, InPalIn. Compared to palliative care, working in intensive care more than doubles the chances of burnout: results from a nationwide comparative study. PLoS One. 2016;11(9):e0162340. https://doi.org/10.1371/journal.pone.0162340.
38. Bowlby J. THE NATURE OF THE CHILD'S TIE TO HIS MOTHER. Int J Psychoanal. 1958;39:350–73.

39. Rottenberg E. "Appendix A. What is at play in play? Derrida's fort/da with freud's fort/da". For the Love of Psychoanalysis. New York: Fordham University Press; 2019. p. 179–89. https://doi.org/10.1515/9780823284139-012.
40. Sheikh FA. Subjectivity, desire and theory: reading Lacan. Cogent Arts Human. 2017;4(129):9565.
41. O'Regan P, Drummond E. Cancer information needs of people with intellectual disability: a review of the literature. Eur J Oncol Nurs. 2008;12(2):142–7. https://doi.org/10.1016/j.ejon.2007.12.001. Epub 2008 Mar 5.

The Models of Mental Growth

7.1 Changes of Comprehension Throughout Children's Growth

Children should be approached according to their own and peculiar level of development. Here, we outline two important ways of doing this. The first is the "theory of mind," i.e., how the child can "enter" in others' minds. This can be helpful in adapting the way we deal with them, in having an idea of how much they are following what we are saying. The second approach is what Jean Piaget proposed about the child's mental development: it will help to distinguish when children's egocentric and non-empathetic behavior becomes broader and open to the dialog.

7.2 Theory of Mind

An important way of communication is the so-called theory of mind. This gives us a key to understand children's mental approach to the others, throughout their growth. The theory of mind is an expression used in philosophy, psychology, and the human sciences to designate the ability to attribute thoughts and intentions to other people (but also to animals or objects). Most neurocognitive theories converge on the following definition: "the ability to make inferences about one's own and other people's mental states" [1]. Here, the word "theory" has mainly the meaning of "conjecture," or better, power of assessment. After childhood, the subjects constantly uses "their" theory of mind, often with the prejudices imposed by the environment; such constant use of the theory of mind is mainly made without being fully aware of it, "intuitively."

Between ages 4 and 5 years, children really start thinking about others' thoughts and feelings (first-order Theory of the Mind), and this is when the true theory of mind emerges. The actual development of the theory of mind generally follows an agreed-upon sequence of steps [2, 3]:

(a) Understanding "wanting." The first step is the realization that others have diverse desires and, to get what they want, people act in different ways.
(b) Understanding "thinking." The second step is the understanding that others also have diverse beliefs about the same thing, and that people's actions are based on what they think is going to happen.
(c) Understanding that "seeing leads to knowing." The third step is recognizing that others have different knowledge approach, and if someone hasn't seen something, they will need extra information to understand.
(d) Understanding "false-beliefs." The fourth step is being aware that others may have false-beliefs that differ from reality, that they can make mistakes.
(e) Understanding "hidden feelings." The final step is being aware that other people can hide their emotions and can feel a different emotion from the one they display.

Second-order Theory of the Mind, which emerges shortly the after first order one (or at age 7) in typically developing children, involves feeling what someone else is thinking or feeling. In addition to second-order Theory of the Mind, higher order cognitive and affective levels involve tasks that require recognizing lies, sarcasm, imagery. These skills typically develop between 8 and 12 years of age [4].

7.3 Piaget's Theories

An important description of children's mental development was done by Jean Piaget (1896–1980), a renowned psychologist of the twentieth century and a pioneer in developmental child psychology. Piaget did not accept the prevailing theory that knowledge was innate or a priori. Instead, he believed a child's knowledge and understanding of the world developed over time, through the child's interaction with the world, and empirically [5]. He explained that at a very young age, children do not have as much empathy as an adult, and have "egocentric thinking," according to their age and abilities. During childhood, a natural cognitive development occurs: children "learn to think," or rather, to experience their environment, becoming aware of their self, and developing their intellectual skills. Piaget's [6] theory maintains that children's intellect and their ability to perceive mature relationships go through specific stages during their development. These stages of children development occur in a fixed order in all children, and in all countries. However, age may vary slightly from child to child.

Piaget proposed four stages of development in children: First—Sensory-motor period (Children 0–2 years), Second—Pre-operational period (Children 2–7 years), Third—Specific period (Children 7–11 years), Fourth—Formal period (Children and adolescents from 11-onward, approximately until they are 19 years old) (see Table 7.1 and Fig. 7.1).

Table 7.1 Piaget's stages of children's development

Sensory Motor Stage (Children 0–2 years) We outline here only few points of this stage, since a rational verbal dialog with the child is impossible here. This stage of children's development is characterized by the child's understanding of the world, coordinating sensory experience with physical action. In this period, there is an advance from innate reflexes to voluntary behaviors. Children at this age have a preference for stimuli that are colorful, bright, with movement and contrast. They repeat events at random, experimenting through their own body. They mainly cry, until they can make other sounds. The first single-word emissions will be around 12 months.
Pre-operational Stage (Children 2–7 years old) Often here appears an important event in the life of a child: schooling (Early Childhood Education). This is a very important social component. The child begins to interact with others, especially with their peers; before this period, relationships were only with their family. Although between 3 and 7 years there is an enormous increase in vocabulary, children during early childhood are governed by "egocentric thinking," this means that the children think according to their individual experiences, so that their thinking is still static, intuitive, and lacking in logic. Therefore, it is common that in this stage they can make mistakes both to interpret an event and to express it. Children at this age will be very curious and want to know, so they will ask their parents the "why" of many things. At this stage, children attribute human thoughts or feelings to objects. This phenomenon is known as animism. Children at this stage of development are unable to put themselves in the shoes of others. That is why children up to the age of 5 do know how to lie but they do not use irony.
Specific period (Children 7–11 years old) Children begin to use logical thinking, but only in concrete situations. In this period, they can perform tasks at a more complex level using logic, as well as perform mathematical operations. However, although they have made a great advance with respect to the pre-logical period, in this period of cognitive development they apply logic with certain limitations: talking about "Here and now" is easier for them. They still do not use abstract thinking and applying on an abstract subject is still complicated for children of this age.
Formal Operations (Children and adolescents 11 years and older) This last period is already characterized by the acquisition of logical reasoning in all circumstances, including abstract reasoning. The novelty in this last period in relation to the child's intelligence is the possibility that they can already make hypotheses about something that they have not learned in a concrete way. Here, learning will begin to be established as a "whole," and not only in a concrete way as in the previous stage.

7.4 How These Models Can Improve the Dialog with the Child About Illness

Being aware of the psychological development of the child is useful to speak appropriately to them. For instance, children do not understand metaphors or irony before the age of 6–7 [7]—two behaviors that entail the capacity to go beyond the literal meaning of a statement—and they cannot reliably distinguish jokes from lies before age 6–7 years [8]. In several children, the theory of mind is not well developed until 8 years of age, and their skills in this area should be assessed [9] before speaking together with them about "serious" problems.

Let's see how this works, when someone talks of health problems.

Piaget's Cognitive Stages of Development

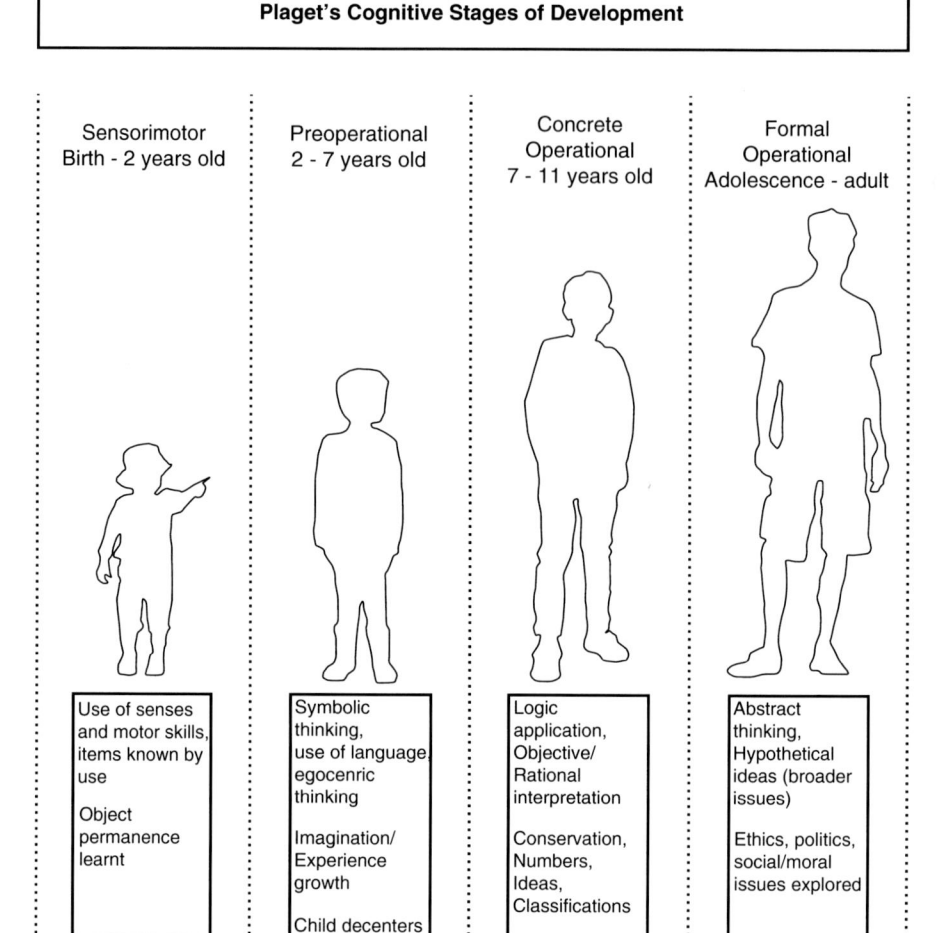

Sensorimotor Birth - 2 years old	Preoperational 2 - 7 years old	Concrete Operational 7 - 11 years old	Formal Operational Adolescence - adult
Use of senses and motor skills, items known by use Object permanence learnt	Symbolic thinking, use of language, egocenric thinking Imagination/ Experience growth Child decenters	Logic application, Objective/ Rational interpretation Conservation, Numbers, Ideas, Classifications	Abstract thinking, Hypothetical ideas (broader issues) Ethics, politics, social/moral issues explored

Fig. 7.1 Stages of children's mental development according to Piaget

Around the age of 5, the concepts of personal death (death applied to oneself) and death unpredictability (the moment of death cannot be known in advance) are acquired. At around 9 years of age, children have a more complete understanding of death.

Between the ages of 4 and 7, children's understanding of the causes of illness is substantially influenced by "magical thinking." Magical thinking is used to describe children's belief that their thoughts, events, or wishes can cause external events (e.g., that illness may be caused by a particular thought or behavior). At the same time, children have an emerging sense of awareness, but little understanding of how diseases spread. This can easily lead to misattribution of the cause, and a feeling of guilt, such as that illness is a punishment for misbehavior [10]. These concepts emphasize the importance of ensuring that the language used with children is

7.4 How These Models Can Improve the Dialog with the Child About Illness

concrete and specific, to avoid misunderstandings or erroneous inferences about the cause of illness [11]. What can we do to promote the communication of the child from 2 to 7 years? We can adjust to their cognitive development level and use the symbolic game: through this activity, many of the children's skills emerge and allow children to form an image of the world. Through play, the roles and situations of the world around them can be interiorized: for instance, that we are doctors and help another person, etc.

Between the ages of 7 and 11 there is a progress in children's understanding of key biological concepts, about the structure and function of the human body and the transmission of diseases. Children at this stage also use their emergent reasoning skills more successfully and approaching more concrete information. For example, they may associate changes such as hair or weight loss with cancer, because they are tangible and observable concepts. A more complete understanding of cancer, chemotherapy or side effects, can become more difficult to understand. What can we do to promote communication in the period from 7 to 11 years? Enhancing their reasoning ability, through questions on specific facts. We can also ask them to help solve questions and ask them questions. For example, "How would you help children who are feeling pain?" "How can we make the nurse arrive when you need them?" "How do we go to Grandma's house if the car is broken?" It is also useful to help them understand the relationships between phenomena that occur in nature or social life: animals, people, time, etc.

In adolescence, there is a substantial influence of the peers [12]; establishing and maintaining group identification can be complicated in these circumstances (pediatric palliative care), due to social isolation caused by long periods of hospital treatment or by feeling or looking different for their life-threatening condition [13]. Adolescence also implies the creation of autonomy from parents or guardians, that could conflict with the need of greater dependency during treatment. The incidence of anxiety, stress disorders, or mood disorders peaks during adolescence [14], making this period one of greatest vulnerability. Recent advances in understanding the maturation of the brain during adolescence are reflected in a shift towards broadening the age range of adolescents to 24 years [15]. Higher order cognitive processes, including executive functions (e.g., inhibitory control, planning, and decision-making) improve during adolescence: there is evidence of a maturation in regions of the prefrontal cortex involved in executive functioning, and cognitive or impulse control capabilities [16, 17]. Adolescents' approach to short-term consequences is particularly relevant in terms of their decision to receive treatments, and can contribute to the tension that is created between their priorities on the one hand, and those of medical care providers on the other (e.g., adolescent's desire for independence and healthcare professional's attention to timely treatment).

What can we do to promote communication in adolescents 11 years and older?

- Try to motivate them to ask questions, use everyday facts and try to reason about the factors that have caused a certain outcome. Help them to make deductions or hypotheses.

- When possible, the help of a reliable friend of the child is useful in vehiculating messages that they would not listen to if expressed by an adult.
- Emotion is important: talking with an adolescent in a familiar setting (familiar music, pets, dresses) can help.

References

1. Schurz M, Perner J. An evaluation of neurocognitive models of theory of mind. Front Psychol. 2015;31;6:1610.
2. Wellman HM, Liu D. Scaling theory of mind tasks. Child Dev. 2004;75:759–63.
3. Wellman HM, Fang F, Peterson CC. Sequential progressions in a theory-of-mind scale: longitudinal perspectives. Child Dev. 2011;82(3):780–92.
4. Westby C, Robinson L. A developmental perspective for promoting theory of mind. Top Lang Disord. 2014;34:362–82. https://doi.org/10.1097/TLD.0000000000000035.
5. Scott HK, Cogburn M. Piaget. In: StatPearls [Internet]. Treasure Island, FL: StatPearls Publishing; 2021.
6. Piaget J. Piaget's theory. In: Mussen P, editor. Handbook of child psychology, vol. 1. 4th ed. New York: Wiley; 1983.
7. Ackerman B. Young children's understanding of a false utterance. Dev Psychol. 1981;31:472–80.
8. Sullivan K, Winner E, Hopfield N. How children tell lie from joke: the role of second order mental state attribution. Br J Dev Psychol. 1995;13:191–204.
9. Calero CI, Salles A, Semelman M, Sigman M. Age and gender dependent development of theory of mind in 6- to 8-years old children. Front Hum Neurosci. 2013;7:281. https://doi.org/10.3389/fnhum.2013.00281.
10. Schonfeld D. Talking with children about death. J Pediatr Health Care. 1993;7(6):269–74.
11. Agrawal J. What do preschool children in India understand about death? An exploratory study. Omega (Westport). 2021;83(2):274–86. https://doi.org/10.1177/0030222819852834. Epub 2019 May 28.
12. Sabramani V, Idris IB, Ismail H, Nadarajaw T, Zakaria E, Kamaluddin MR. Bullying and its associated individual, peer, family and school factors: evidence from Malaysian National Secondary School students. Int J Environ Res Public Health. 2021;18(13):7208. https://doi.org/10.3390/ijerph18137208.
13. Ingersgaard MV, Fridh MK, Thorsteinsson T, Adamsen L, Schmiegelow K, Baekgaard Larsen H. A qualitative study of adolescent cancer survivors perspectives on social support from healthy peers—a RESPECT study. J Adv Nurs. 2021;77(4):1911–20. https://doi.org/10.1111/jan.14732. Epub 2021 Jan 20
14. Solmi M, Radua J, Olivola M, Croce E, Soardo L, de Pablo GS, Il Shin J, Kirkbride JB, Jones P, Kim JH, Kim JY, Carvalho AF, Seeman MV, Correll CU, Fusar-Poli P. Age at onset of mental disorders worldwide: large-scale meta-analysis of 192 epidemiological studies. Mol Psychiatry. 2021;27:281–95. https://doi.org/10.1038/s41380-021-01161-7. Epub ahead of print.
15. Backes EP, Bonnie RJ, editors. The promise of adolescence realizing opportunity for all youth. Washington, DC: National Academies Press (US); 2019.
16. Crone EA, Steinbeis N. Neural perspectives on cognitive control development during childhood and adolescence. Trends Cogn Sci. 2017;21(3):205–15.
17. Steinberg L. Cognitive and affective development in adolescence. Trends Cogn Sci. 2005;9:69.

Part III

Advocates of the Child Who Cannot Speak

Treating those children and babies who cannot talk is a paradigm for treating those who know how to express themselves. If you become skilled in talking to them and communicating your ideas, senses, diagnoses, warnings, smartness, you enter a world you could not imagine before, but you also become more able to understand the needs and hopes and symptoms of those who can talk. Nonetheless, speech is a unique human quality, it identifies the human being. That is a matter of fact, but produces the risk of not considering totally human those who cannot speak. This is an unconscious inference (though theorized by philosophers), and can lead to malpractice. Here, we will see how, on the converse, babies and children who do not speak preserve their human dignity, but also how they can communicate, and how we can help them in doing it.

The Respect Due and Denied to Those Who Lack Speech

8.1 The Human Strength of the Speech

Language has a supreme importance for humans. Its first aim is expressing emotions [1, 2]. It is also an important step in psychological growth. For Jaques Lacan, the emerging of the language signs the end of the oral phase of human primordial libido, represented by breast suction. As human beings, our very subjectivity is defined by language. As Emile Benveniste puts it, humans cannot be imagined without language: even though we are inclined to imagine a primordial time when a man discovered another one and between the two of them language was created little by little, this is not what happened [3]. "We can never get back to man separated from language and we shall never see him inventing it. It is a speaking man whom we find in the world, a man speaking to another man, and language provides the very definition of man" [4]. Anyway, several types of language exist: for instance, the language of the body, through which the unconscious often expresses itself; "it speaks where it hurts," Lacan said, to describe the non-verbal language of the psychosomatic alarms thrown by our depth. All this means that language is a basic element for personhood.

In conclusion, when a spoken language is not possible, other forms exist, and should be facilitated and supported. These forms should be detected when they are hidden and difficult to spot. Communication and language can have peculiar ways and peculiar times and can get many forms. Babies have forms of protolanguage that allow them to communicate in a non-verbal mode; disabled children can communicate in their own way, and tools exist to facilitate this. Communication and language are possible for everyone, any child has its way of communicating. The risk is that the inability to communicate verbally might produce diffidence, isolation, and finally discrimination.

© The Author(s), under exclusive license to Springer Nature Switzerland AG 2022
C. V. Bellieni, *A New Holistic-Evolutive Approach to Pediatric Palliative Care*, https://doi.org/10.1007/978-3-030-96256-2_8

8.2 Mentally Impaired Children

Mentally disabled children have a communicative barrier since their way of expressing their feelings and wishes is not the common one. The risk is that someone may infer from this difference a personhood difference, a lower dignity. People with a mental disability are in the group of non-verbal patients because they speak in ways other than by words, or use words in an uncommon way. The status of verbal patients opens to a chance for a better treatment, but the right to a good treatment is a universal right, and the barriers of speech should be overcome when dealing with non-verbal children, to give everybody the same level of health care. Nonetheless, this can be deficient. Taking care of those who can speak is easier than those patients with mental disabilities, whose symptoms and needs can be deduced sometimes from their mimics or movements. Interpreting symptoms is hard if a patient is not overtly collaborative, and several doctors are not able or do not want to invest time in doing it. An unfair matter lies at the base of the distance between non-verbal patients and appropriate care: it is the unconscious reluctance in considering completely human those who are overtly different from the average people, and the lack of speech in the patient is an alibi for a lack of caregivers' communication efforts. According to some philosophers, only what can be rationally spoken is real (Ludwig Wittgenstein, in [5]): for the rationalist philosopher Ludwig Wittgenstein, the reality is subordinated to the words through which we describe it; and if there is no word to describe a phenomenon, it simply does not exist or, as he wrote in his Tractatus Logico-Philosophicus, "Whereof one cannot speak, thereof one must be silent" (1921). Nonetheless, much of life happens under the tag of silence or of non-verbal communication; silence can be a communicative tool and non-verbal communication can find several ways to express our ideas in a comprehensible way. The problem consists in finding the ways to understand a non-verbal patient, as we will describe later.

An intriguing article was recently published on the situation of disabled people, under the unequivocable title: "Canada is plunging towards a human rights disaster for disabled people" describing a worrying scenario where the services of end of life can become "a substitute for the care that could make his life livable (…). The alternate offer, of a medically assisted death, shows how well-meaning policies can excuse inadequate care" [6]. And another recent paper denounces: "Oregon Hospitals Didn't Have Shortages. So Why Were Disabled People Denied Care?" [7]. This is overtly alarming. And the first step in this discriminative scenario is the incapacity of caregivers to listen to people with mental disability. Thus, mentally disabled or comatose children may receive less appropriate palliative care because they are far from the idea of someone who can be described with words or who can describe their illness with words. Only in 2020 the official definition of the word "pain" has changed to include those who cannot describe with words their suffering [8]. Until that date, this definition made by the International Association for the Study of Pain (IASP) was: "An unpleasant sensory and emotional experience associated with actual or potential tissue damage, or described in terms of such damage" [9]. The prerequisite for pain in this definition was to be described with words. Then it was transformed into the following: "An unpleasant sensory and emotional experience associated with, or resembling that associated with, actual or potential tissue damage," [10] followed by this comment: "Verbal description is only one of several behaviors to express pain; inability to communicate does not negate the possibility that a human or a nonhuman animal experiences pain" [10]. It is easy to understand that mentally disabled children, who are intrinsically irrational and whose needs they cannot describe with simple words as the other children, are out of sight in the contemporary era, they are "mostly invisible to the Healthcare System" [11] being not considered full persons [12, 13] or full patients.

8.3 Perinatal Patients

The initial state of the human life requires smartness and capacity for empathy to treat it like any other state of life. It is a big flaw to think that since a human being does not look like a human being, since they do not yet have all the structures of a human being including voice, then they are not a human being, and should not be treated as a human being. Instead, they are humans, and *it is possible* to treat them as a human being: feeding them, healing them, soothing them and, also providing them palliative care [14]. But the lack of speech is evident in newborns, a human feature that would have enrolled them among humans with no hesitation, if present. The lack of speech can be the alibi for a different treatment.

Nonetheless, we can treat newborns with all the best medical tools we use for adults: tools for resuscitation, brain damage prevention, antibiotic therapy, and much more. Today, we can even treat fetuses by temporarily extracting them from the uterus without cutting the umbilical cord that gives them nutrition and oxygen, that is, making them "born" momentarily; then putting them back in the uterus, closing it up, and giving birth to them a second time, when the pregnancy comes to term [15]. We also observe fetuses recognized as patients during prenatal surgery, because several of them are more developed than some preterm babies [16, 17]. The moral or physical distinction between late-term fetuses and preterm newborns is really ambiguous and hard to sustain. This is why perinatal palliative care features very preterm babies and starts with the prenatal diagnosis.

Several philosophers argue that newborns and toddlers cannot be described as "persons," because they lack several human features, such as self-consciousness, speech, and autonomy [18]; Daniel Roger and colleagues so expressed: "It is commonly argued that a serious right to life is grounded only in actual, relatively advanced psychological capacities a being has acquired. Increasingly it is being argued that such accounts also entail the permissibility of infanticide, with several proponents of these theories accepting this consequence. We show, however, that these accounts imply the permissibility of even more unpalatable acts than infanticide performed on infants: organ harvesting, live experimentation, sexual interference, and discriminatory killing" [19]. The philosophical dilemma of treating as humans those who do not appear humans, is a very old conundrum. And the problem is great in the early stages of life, when human characteristics are not yet evident [20]. It can be thought that being human means having certain characteristics, for example, self-awareness, that newborns don't have. But neither common people have them during sleep, and that does not mean they cease being human: it is not our phenomenic characteristics that give us the identity of men or women.

"Homo est et qui est futurus" (transl. "Human is who will be it") wrote Tertullian in the second century AC; nonetheless, it seems too simplistic to say that something is something simply because it will be that. I may have the idea of my future child, but the idea is not a child just because they will be. Yet Tertullian continues in his treatise: "etiam fructus omnis iam in semine est" ("all the fruit is already present in the seed") and this is the point: in their essence, the fruit and the tree have no differences with the seed but in their form. The seed is small and certainly does not look like the fruit or the tree, but it has their substance, their essence: just let it develop and it will become a tree, it will be a fruit, because it already is. Today, we give this identity a name: DNA. In the small seed, there is the same code as in the huge oak which it will become; in the newborn, there is the same unique and unrepeatable code that will be present in the adult whom it will become. Newborns are small, immobile, mute, they are more similar in size to small pets than to humans, but they are human.

Some factors push to deny this identity. First, the instinct of preserving ourselves from stress. This pushes to consider the newborn baby different from a full person because they have a high mortality rate and the loss, death, disappearance of a full person is terrible: it is better not to consider them persons in so far as they can die. There will be time to love them if they survive! This has been a criterion for centuries, when infanticide was considered a minor crime, a crime against the lineage and not against the person. And this prejudice still persists: until the end of the 90s of the last century, most doctors maintained that the newborns were not persons; that they did not feel pain; and at the beginning of this century still many European pediatricians argued that in case of future disability it is better for the newborn to die, basing this decision not on the will to do the best interest of the child [21, 22], even though many disabled people accept their disability, and we cannot know at birth if this child will accept it or not. This is also argued to be in the interests of the parents who are presumed to live better without—instead than with—the disabled child. The American philosopher Peter Singer affirms the liceity in eliminating a disabled baby so that parents can have a "replacement" child after the death of the former [23]. And several neonatal resuscitation guidelines are based on the principle of resuscitating (or not) according to parents' wishes [24, 25]; this would not happen in the case of an adult patient: you do not choose about an husband's life according to the interests of his wife, or vice versa.

Second, it has been argued that newborns are different from the adult because the adult behaves unlike a newborn. It is said that somebody is a person when they have the capacity to decide, speak, and choose; of course, babies don't have it. But this is not what makes a person become a person. As Severinus Boethius (fifth century AC) said, the person is "Individua substantia naturae rationalis," that is, to be a person it is necessary to have a rational nature, that is, not to be rational, but to belong to the human gender that is rational in its nature; and it is necessary to be an individual.

This is the case of newborns, and also the case of comatose patients: they are individuals and belong to the human gender; the fact that they momentaneously lack of consciousness or of other evident human qualities does not mean that they are not human.

References

1. Doyle CM, Lindquist KA. When a word is worth a thousand pictures: Language shapes perceptual memory for emotion. J Exp Psychol Gen. 2018;147(1):62–73
2. Torre JD, Lieberman MD: Putting feeling into words: Affect labeling as implicit emotion regulation. Emotion Review. 2018;10(2):116–124
3. Laufer L, Santos B. Language and vulnerability—a lacanian analysis of respect. Front Psychol. 2017;8:2279.
4. Benveniste E. Subjectivity in language. In: Verstraeten P, Ruwet N, editors. Problems in general linguistics. Coral Gables, FL: University Miami Press; 1963/1967. p. 223–30.
5. Loizzo J. Intersubjectivity in Wittgenstein and Freud: other minds and the foundations of psychiatry. Theor Med. 1997;18(4):379–400. https://doi.org/10.1023/a:1005769707626.
6. Braswell H. Canada is plunging toward a human rights disaster for disabled people. The Washington Post. 2021.
7. Shapiro J. Oregon hospitals didn't have shortages. So why were disabled people denied care? Npr News. 2020.
8. Raja SN, Carr DB, Cohen M, Finnerup NB, Flor H, Gibson S, Keefe FJ, Mogil JS, Ringkamp M, Sluka KA, Song XJ, Stevens B, Sullivan MD, Tutelman PR, Ushida T, Vader K. The revised International Association for the Study of Pain definition of pain: concepts, challenges, and compromises. Pain. 2020;161(9):1976–82.
9. Merskey H. Logic, truth and language in concepts of pain. Qual Life Res. 1994;3(Suppl 1):S69–76. https://doi.org/10.1007/BF00433379.
10. International Association for the Studies of Pain. IASP Announces Revised Definition of Pain. 2020. https://www.iasp-pain.org/publications/iasp-news/iasp-announces-revised-definition-of-pain/
11. The Lancet (Editorial) Learning disability: a cause for shame. Lancet. 2008;372(9637):420.
12. Agmon M, Sa'ar A, Araten-Bergman T. The person in the disabled body: a perspective on culture and personhood from the margins. Int J Equity Health. 2016;15(1):147. https://doi.org/10.1186/s12939-016-0437-2.
13. Blain S, McKeever P. Revealing personhood through biomusic of individuals without communicative interaction ability. Augment Altern Commun. 2011;27(1):1–4. https://doi.org/10.310 9/07434618.2011.556663.
14. Berry SN. Providing palliative care to neonates with anencephaly in the home setting. J Hosp Palliat Nurs. 2021;23(4):367–74. https://doi.org/10.1097/NJH.0000000000000770.
15. Lopyan NM, Perrone EE, Gadepalli SK, Raval MV, Tsao K, Rich BS, American Academy of Pediatrics Section on Surgery Delivery of Surgical Care Committee. Current status of subspecialization in pediatric surgery: a focus on fetal surgery. J Pediatr Surg. 2021;57(4):610–5. https://doi.org/10.1016/j.jpedsurg.2021.05.008. Epub ahead of print.
16. Chervenak FA, McCullough LB. Ethical dimensions of the fetus as a patient. Best Pract Res Clin Obstet Gynaecol. 2017;43:2–9. https://doi.org/10.1016/j.bpobgyn.2016.12.007. Epub 2017 Jan 23.
17. William PR, Kaufmann CL. Fetus as patient—medical legal and ethical dimensions. J Fla Med Assoc. 1983;70(9):764–7.
18. Tännsjö T. Should parents of neonates with bleak prognosis be encouraged to opt for another child with better odds? On the notion of moral replaceability. Pediatrics. 2018;142(Suppl 1):S552–7. https://doi.org/10.1542/peds.2018-0478F.

19. Rodger D, Blackshaw BP, Miller C. Beyond infanticide: how psychological accounts of persons can justify harming infants. New Bioeth. 2018;24(2):106–21. https://doi.org/10.1080/20502877.2018.1438771. Epub 2018 Feb 21.
20. Andaya E, Campo-Engelstein L. Conceptualizing pain and personhood in the periviable period: perspectives from reproductive health and neonatal intensive care unit clinicians. Soc Sci Med. 2021;269:113558. https://doi.org/10.1016/j.socscimed.2020.113558. Epub 2020 Nov 29
21. Brick C, Kahane G, Wilkinson D, Caviola L, Savulescu J. Worth living or worth dying? The views of the general public about allowing disabled children to die. J Med Ethics. 2020;46(1):7–15. https://doi.org/10.1136/medethics-2019-105639. Epub 2019 Oct 15.
22. Rebagliato M, Cuttini M, Broggin L, Berbik I, de Vonderweid U, Hansen G, Kaminski M, Kollée LA, Kucinskas A, Lenoir S, Levin A, Persson J, Reid M, Saracci R, EURONIC Study Group (European Project on Parents' Information and Ethical Decision Making in Neonatal Intensive Care Units). Neonatal end-of-life decision making: physicians' attitudes and relationship with self-reported practices in 10 European countries. JAMA. 2000;284(19):2451–9. https://doi.org/10.1001/jama.284.19.2451.
23. Kemmerer LA. Peter Singer on expendability. Between the Species. 2007;7:10.
24. Janvier A, Barrington KJ, Aziz K, Bancalari E, Batton D, Bellieni C, Bensouda B, Blanco C, Cheung PY, Cohn F, Daboval T, Davis P, Dempsey E, Dupont-Thibodeau A, Ferretti E, Farlow B, Fontana M, Fortin-Pellerin E, Goldberg A, Hansen TW, Haward M, Kovacs L, Lapointe A, Lantos J, Morley C, Moussa A, Musante G, Nadeau S, O'Donnell CP, Orfali K, Payot A, Ryan CA, Sant'anna G, Saugstad OD, Sayeed S, Stokes TA, Verhagen E. CPS position statement for prenatal counselling before a premature birth: simple rules for complicated decisions. Paediatr Child Health. 2014;19(1):22–4.
25. Lamau MC, Ruiz E, Merrer J, Sibiude J, Huon C, Lepercq J, Goffinet F, Jarreau PH. A new individualized prognostic approach to the management of women at risk of extreme preterm birth in France: effect on neonatal outcome. Arch Pediatr. 2021;28(5):366–73. https://doi.org/10.1016/j.arcped.2021.04.005. Epub 2021 May 28.

The Communicative Features of Non-verbal Patients

9.1 Sensoriality and Pain in the Newborn

We have seen that pediatric palliative care can find an important obstacle when communication is lacking. Of course, babies in their first years of life, and in particular newborns, seem to be relatively unreactive and unresponsive; or their reactions are considered generical or not aimed to a scope o to a communication, consequently they receive no communication from the bystanders. Here, we show the way newborns can understand and be aware of the surrounding world.

9.1.1 Sense Development

The human being develops a set of brain and peripheral structures to be able to feel external stimuli, and this set already works since mid-pregnancy. Even before birth, the subject can receive sound, tactile, gustatory, and painful stimuli that will have two functions: first, to mold their nervous system; second, to prepare them for the life that awaits them outside the uterus [1]. Modeling the nervous system means pruning those excessive and useless groups of neurons that are destined to disappear; and the stimuli for this pruning are precisely the stimuli that come from outside [2]. The uterus is not a safe but a filter: a safe does not allow anything to pass through its walls, while a filter allows only what is useful to pass through. Noises from the external environment pass through this filter, as well as the mother's voice, so that the fetus after birth will be able to recognize them: several experiments have shown this [3, 4]. Through this filter, the flavors of the things that the mother eats pass, and arrive through the mother's blood to the amniotic fluid: during pregnancy, the fetus continuously sucks [5] the amniotic fluid flavored by the taste of the things the mother eats. This is how our food preferences are formed, with the imprint on our brain of those flavors that we feel before we are born. Odors pass through this filter, as do flavors [6]: at the base of the fetal brain, there is a small organ called the vomeronasal organ that is used to perceive odors, particularly those of fluids [7]. So the stimuli that arrive to the fetus shape its brain but also prepare it for the external world: at birth, the little ones will be able to look for breast milk, because they have already known its taste and smell before birth; and they will be able to search for their mother because they already know her voice [8]. These notes extracted from the prenatal studies are important for the newborns: their senses are well structured, they can be aware of the presence of their mother, of her voice and smell, when they are in her arms. The skin-to-skin contact has an important influx on their well-being, as well as the sweet taste of milk that they adore. Their mother's voice can calm them, and the voice of a foreign person can harm them as well. Their capability of perceiving the environment is well structured, and the harm that a noisy room can provoke on them is evident. The presence of a developed amygdala, the center of stress elaboration, allow them feel anxiety and stress as well.

9.1.2 The Sense of Pain

Like the other senses, pain also develops from mid-pregnancy. In mid-pregnancy, the fetus—and the preterm newborn—gets the nerves that carry painful stimuli to the spinal cord, and from the spinal cord to the brain. In the brain, the painful stimulus is processed by the thalamus, which, even when the cerebral cortex is still immature, is sufficient to decrypt pain signals [9]. Obviously, all these sensations will not be conscious [10], as they will not be accompanied by the ability to realize them, to describe them, to understand their origin; however, these sensations are present, strong, well perceived, also in the precociously born preterm baby (Fig. 9.1).

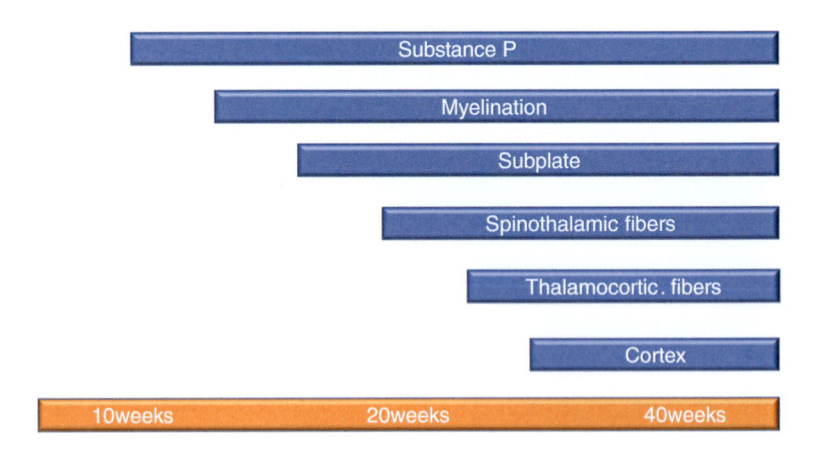

Fig. 9.1 The appearance of the structures used by the nervous system to make the baby feel pain

9.2 Communication Skills of the Babies

9.2.1 The Newborn

It is a matter of fact that babies in their first stages of life can communicate. This kind of communication can be considered a form of protolanguage and can be exploited to communicate with the baby and to become aware of their skills and wishes.

For one of the pioneers of the neonatal care, Heidi Als, even preterm babies are "psychobiologically social" [11], and she developed all her strategy of intervention on the signs and hints that a baby can express. She called it "Neonatal Individual Developmental Care Assessment Program" [12], and it was the way to reckon from specific signals the needs of a mute preterm baby, divided into several subsystems (autonomous system, relationships, etc.); when, thanks to the baby's signals, a specific subsystem is acknowledged to require attention, a tailored care is started. This system gives an important improvement to babies' neurological and developmental outcomes.

Thus, it is not true that a newborn or a toddler cannot communicate. The problem is that they do it in their specific way. What is needed is our attention. The analgesic strategy called "sensorial saturation," which we will deal with later on, has been developed with this aim [13, 14]. Watching the responses of the babies to several gentle interventions performed during a painful maneuver such as a heel-prick, it was seen that message, gentle speaking, giving oral sugar relaxed the baby so much that they did not feel the pain produced by the heel lancing. The sign we should wait for is babies' regular sucking: this is the signal of complete relaxation when the analgesia provided is at its maximum level: this is a way of communicative success.

The newborns also express their feelings with other aspects of their behavior. Their crying, for instance. Crying is not specific enough to say that a newborn is feeling pain, but its features can be exploited to assess the level of pain they are feeling. In other words, when a baby is crying, we can infer that they are feeling pain only if this is confirmed by contextual-environmental data, as there is no specific pain-crying [15]; but crying has some characteristics, namely its pitch, its rhythm, and its continuity in time, that dramatically change above a certain threshold of pain, and this can be used to score pain [16]. In other words, we cannot unveil the reason they are crying, but they can "tell" the level of stress they are going through. Similar results were found by other researchers who described neonatal crying as a form of protolanguage [17].

Newborns also have several ways to manifest stress: hiccup, vomiting, sudden skin color changes. These are expression of distress, and spasmodic movements or hypertone are a message of extreme suffering and anxiety. But they can also send messages of relaxation when they feel our gentle touch, when we are taking care of them, as a form of communicating their ease. This is summed up in Table 9.1.

Table 9.1 Communicative signs of the baby

Communication of relax:
• Normal skin color
• Arms and legs flexed or tucked
• Hand touching his face
• Hand to mouth or in mouth
• Sucking
• Looking at you
• Smiling and looks relaxed
• Regular breathing rate
• If your baby is on a monitor, regular heartbeat
Communication of stress:
• Hiccupping
• Yawning
• Sneezing
• Frowning
• Looking away
• Squirming
• Frantic, disorganized activity
• Arms and legs pushing away
• Arms and legs limp and floppy
• Skin color changes

9.2.2 The Toddler

Even the pre-verbal children have the opportunity of expressing themselves, with a sort of protolanguage. Allowing children to express themselves and trying to understand their communication is also important at an early stage, which can be defined as pre-verbal. In fact, infants' mimic expressions have the place of their words, as words will appear later. In particular, two extreme expressions have a strong impact on communication: laughing and crying. Both cause self-reassurance and self-comfort in the child, and have a strong unmistakable impact on the viewer, as a message of joy or pain. These two extreme expressions are flanked in this mimic language by two other more nuanced expressions: the pout and the smile, which give a less dramatic but always very explicit message [18].

In this epoch of their life, children's expressive abilities evolve improving their expressive skills. Fern Sussman described this evolution in four main steps [19]. They are: the *Own Agenda Stage*, the *Requester Stage*, the *Early Communicator Stage*, and the *Partner Stage*. Children in the *Own Agenda Stage* do not understand how they can influence the people around them by addressing an idea directly to the bystanders, which makes their communication predominantly pre-intentional. Their interactions with others are usually short and minimalist. Parents discern how and what babies are feeling by observing their gestures, body movements, smiles, and screams. At the *Requester Stage*, children begin to realize that their actions can affect others. They begin communicating their needs to parents by pulling or guiding them to objects, areas, or games they love. In the *Early Communicator Stage*, the child's communication lasts longer and becomes more intentional. They may begin to repeat some of the things they feel to communicate their needs to others.

Slowly, the child begins a two-way interaction, indicating the things they want to show their parents. In the *Partner Stage*, the child becomes a more effective communicator. While not all babies go through all four stages in a specific order, many tend to start at their *own agenda stage* and progress through the requester and *early communicator stages*, eventually reaching the *partner stage* as their age progresses [20].

Pre-linguistic skills can be used intentionally to communicate one's needs, or involuntarily. These typically develop around 9–15 months of age and lay the foundations for language [21, 22], and emotional development [23].

Turn-taking is a salient pre-linguistic skill that lays the foundation for communication and self-regulation skills in children, thus contributing to subsequent language development [24, 25]. Taking turns is an important part of communication development for young children. When children learn to take turns, they learn the basic rhythm of communication that back-and-forth exchange between people.

Another important pre-linguistic skill is eye contact: as a part of normal communication, children involve eye contact with parents [26].

All this has its real importance. It is necessary to overcome the prejudice that, in the absence of a verbal language, the subjects cannot express themselves and, not knowing how to express themselves, they should not be listened to. This mistake would be fatal in pediatric palliative care. Parents and caregivers may believe that their children should at least speak correctly, smile upon request, or perform some specific skill, before accepting them as part of their family or interacting with them; but how many hints and signs and symptoms are expressed by the child and we are not noticing it! And how many children are misdiagnosed for this, ranging from errors in pain assessment, to a kaleidoscope of possible mistakes.

9.3 Communication Strategies for Mentally Disabled Children

Children with complex communication needs may have impairments in language production and/or comprehension [27], resulting from different etiologies such as cerebral palsy, Down syndrome, developmental disabilities, or speech-language impairment. Recent studies have revealed that people with complex communication needs often face barriers in expressing and/or understanding emotions and may have fewer opportunities to talk and learn about their own emotions [28, 29].

Children with complex communication needs often present some challenges in expressing emotions, not only via linguistic modes of communication (e.g., difficult to produce speech or to access vocabulary that enables them to understand and express emotions), but also in non-linguistic modalities (e.g., motor and/or sensory difficulties). Therefore, their communication partners may face difficulties in identifying, interpreting, and discussing emotions with a child [29] and may overestimate or underestimate the child's emotional experience [30]. As a result, the need of learning emotional language of children with complex communication needs can be challenging, but also ignored.

Augmentative and Alternative Communication is the set of knowledge, techniques, strategies, and technologies that facilitate and increase communication in people who have difficulty using the most common communication channels, in particular oral language and writing [31]. The adjective "Augmentative" indicates that it is aimed not at replacing, but at increasing natural communication: the objective of this intervention must be the expansion of communication skills through all the available methods and channels: vocalizations, verbal language residue, gestures, and signs. Augmentative and Alternative Communication is therefore not a substitute for oral language, nor does it inhibit its development when it can emerge; it is always a support to relationship, understanding, and thinking. Today, we tend not to use the adjective "Alternative" because it seems supplanting the existing methods of communication. There is a significant body of evidence on the benefits of Augmentative and Alternative Communication in supporting the language and communication development of children with complex communication needs [32]. Children with developmental delay have problems with both receptive language (i.e., understanding the use of others' symbols) and expressive language (i.e., producing symbols to share with others). Augmentative and Alternative Communication can act favorably on both these fronts, if it is used appropriately [33, 34].

Augmentative and Alternative Communication was born in the 1970s in Canada and the United States, especially in the context of infantile cerebral palsy or disorders with prevalent expressive difficulty [35]; it was structured in the 1980s, with the establishment of the International Augmentative and Alternative Communication Society, a mixed association of professionals, users, and family members, through which it began to spread throughout the world and in particular in English-speaking countries. In parallel, it began to broaden its scope of intervention to mental retardation, other disabilities with associated communication disorders and severe language comprehension disorders. Augmentative and Alternative Communication is indicated for every person who has complex communication needs with a receptive, expressive, motor, cognitive, and visual linguistic component. Disability conditions that may require Augmentative and Alternative Communication interventions include congenital, acquired, developmental, and temporary neurological conditions.

Augmentative and Alternative Communication can be unassisted and assisted. By augmentative and alternative non-assisted communication, we mean that communication that does not require the use of external devices to communicate, because it uses the skills of the individual himself: facial expressions, vocalizations, gestures, signs, and residual verbal language. Augmentative and Alternative Assisted Communication, on the converse, uses external devices for communication, which can be electronic (low or high technology) or non-electronic. Non-electronic devices include symbol or image systems, communication tables, visual activity patterns. Low-tech electronic devices include voice communication aids (such as Vocal Output Communication Aids—VOCA) that play individual messages or sequential messages for a few minutes. High-tech electronic devices include complex aids: multi-box symbolic communicators with interchangeable faceplates for voice output; alphabetic communicators and dynamic displays (Fig. 9.2).

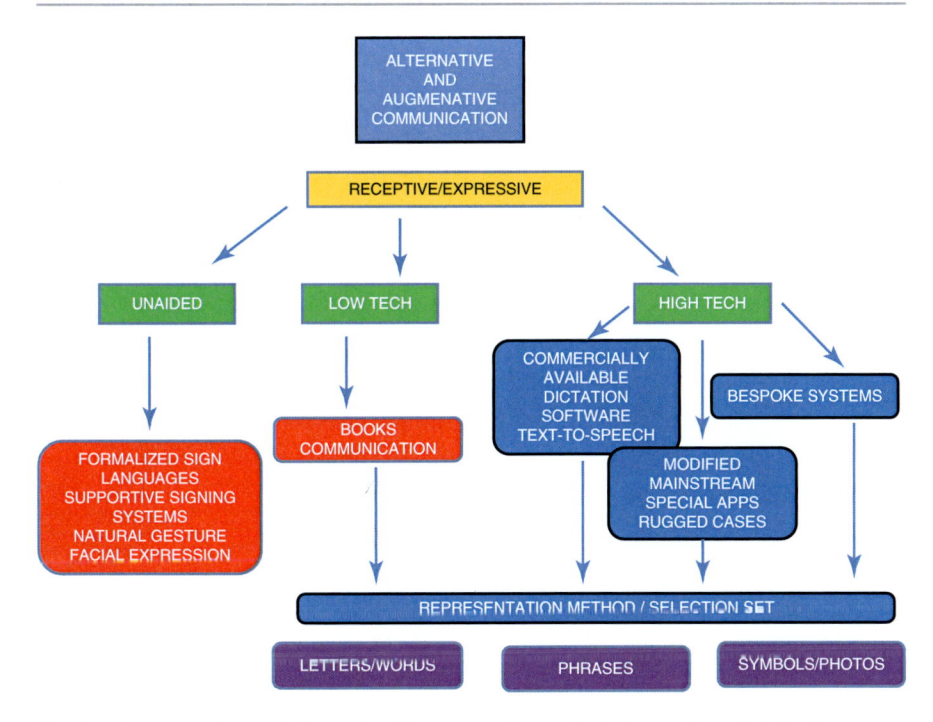

9.3 Communication Strategies for Mentally Disabled Children

Fig. 9.2 Augmentative and Alternative Communication tools. (Adapted from Ref. [36])

There are no minimum prerequisites necessary to use this type of communication, so there is neither a minimum cognitive level, and there is no level of severity of the disability, nor an age below which it is not recommended to start. Obviously, the collaboration and committment by the rehabilitation services are needed.

Augmentative and Alternative Communication includes communication systems such as sign language, speech output devices, and image exchange; these systems have actually been shown to improve different subjects' skills such as social skills, modify and improve behaviors, and above all better learning. Among the tools available are communication books. A communication book is a form of Augmentative and Alternative Communication that allows the user to communicate by pointing or looking at specific sections of various pages. Communication books often contain images or image symbols accompanied by a word or label [37].

The Picture Exchange Communication System (PECS) is one of the Augmentative and Alternative Communication systems used most frequently by individuals with autism, this system includes six phases (Table 9.2).

PECS has been tested favorably in individuals with autism [38] and with multiple disabilities [39]. Portable devices (tablets, smart phones, etc.) are becoming more and more ubiquitous in society and researchers have begun to enjoy the effects of AAC systems in improving social, academic, and communicative activities [40, 41].

Table 9.2 The phases of the PECS

Phase I, the child makes a request through the exchange of images, that is, the child indicates or gives a figure depicting the preferred element to a communicative partner, then the child receives the element.
Phase II, the same procedures as Phase I, but the distance between the child and the communicative partner has increased and the child has to move to give the partner the image.
Phase III, there is no partner, and the child is taught to discriminate between multiple symbols on a communication book.
Phase IV involves teaching the child to use a sentence structure with an image of "I want."
Phase V, the child is taught to answer questions like "What do you want?"
Phase VI, the child is taught how to answer other questions like "What do you like?"

9.3.1 Pain Assessment in Mentally Disabled Children

It is important to reckon that in mentally disabled people, pain can be assessed with specific tools, because it is evident that they cannot use a common VAS scale. The assessment of pain in a person with an intellectual disability is often difficult and complicated. The person with an intellectual disability may be unable to verbally communicate their discomfort. For the carer, who knows the individual with an intellectual disability, knowing how they usually respond to painful stimuli helps to detect new instances of pain. The health professionals in an emergency department, unlikely have met before people with an intellectual disability, and therefore detecting pain by observing their behavior or using self-report measures gets hard. There have been some attempts to categorize behavioral responses to pain by people with an intellectual disability; however, emergency nurses/doctors must also rely on the person who knows and accompanies the patient with an intellectual disability [42].

Tools to assess non-verbally communicating children's pain exist, and the NCCPC-PV [43] seems to be the easiest to use for pain assessment in cognitively impaired children [44]. NCCPC-PV is the acronym for Non-communicating Children's Pain Checklist—Postoperative Version. It is evident that a single feature, often associated with pain, such as crying or grimace, is not sufficient to assess pain, for its lack of sensibility and specificity [45]. Therefore, this kind of scales integrates multiple items, gives each one a score, and obtains a final score by the sum of the single items' scores. In Table 9.3, we report the NCCPC scale.

9.4 Communicating with Children with Disabilities

In pediatric palliative care, it is important to be utterly aware that anyone can communicate; the way they can do it will be personal and subordinated to their health state and mental development. Anyway, children with disabilities are to be considered communicating patients, and if we cannot communicate with them, it is not their fault; it is a tenet to improve our communications skills with these patients. Children with mental disabilities are part of our community, it is imperative trying to communicate with them. It can seem hard to get; yet, when you are familiar with their

9.4 Communicating with Children with Disabilities

Table 9.3 Non-communicating Children's Pain Checklist—Postoperative Version

Vocal
  Moaning, whining, whimpering (fairly soft)
  Crying (moderately loud)
  Screaming/yelling (very loud)
  A specific sound or word for pain (e.g., a word, cry, or type of laugh)

Social
  Not cooperating, cranky, irritable, unhappy
  Less interaction with others, withdrawn
  Seeking comfort or physical closeness
  Being difficult to distract, not able to satisfy or pacify

Facial
  A furrowed brow
  A change in eyes, including: squinching of eyes, eyes opened wide, eyes frowning
  Turning down of mouth, not smiling
  Lips puckering up, tight, pouting, or quivering
  Clenching or grinding teeth, chewing, or thrusting tongue out

Activity
  Not moving, less active, quiet
  Jumping around, agitated, fidgety

Body and limbs
  Floppy
  Stiff, spastic, tense, rigid
  Gesturing to or touching part of the body that hurts
  Protecting, favoring, or guarding part of the body that hurts
  Flinching or moving the body part away, being sensitive to touch
  Moving the body in a specific way to show pain (e.g., head back, arms down, curls up)

Physiological
  Shivering
  Changing in color, pallor
  Sweating, perspiring
  Tears
  Sharp intake of breath, gasping
  Breath holding

Each item should receive a 0–3 score, according to the frequency it is present (from never to very often). The sum of the single scores gives a final assessment. A total score of 11 or more indicates a child has moderate to severe pain. Based on unpublished data from this same sample, a total score of 6–10 indicates a child has mild pain

parents, you soon understand they communicate with their child, even in the worst health conditions [46]. Thus, it is our prejudice what moves us away from the idea of communicating with the mentally disabled child. In a recent study [47], 20 physicians involved in the care of disabled people were interviewed about their difficulties and experiences in communication with their patients. Concerns coalesced around four broad categories: communication experiences with people who are deaf or have impaired hearing, communication with people who are blind or have vision impairment, communication with people who have intellectual disabilities, and recommendations for improving communication. The conclusion was that communicating with patients with intellectual disabilities raised particular concerns: participants often preferred to interact with caregivers and did minimal efforts to involve patients.

It is also important to give these patients the same opportunities we give to the whole population. For instance, distraction while waiting for a test should be provided either through videogames or through the presence of their parents [48].

Nurses and doctors pay attention to the protection of the mentally retarded individual's health; they should identify and treat their ailments. But because of the disability of the child, a lack of communication and obstacles in the exchange and interpretation of information could take place between the health professional and the mentally retarded child. Thus, when necessary, nurses and doctors have the responsibility of facilitating effective communication since the mentally retarded individuals are not always capable of speaking [49]. Here in Table 9.4, we report some hints that can be useful in this task.

Table 9.4 Hints to interact with people with disabilities [50]

Speak Directly
Use clear simple communications. Most people, whether or not they have a mental health disability, appreciate it. If someone is having difficulty processing sounds or information, as often occurs in psychiatric disorders, your message is more apt to be clearly understood. Speak directly to the person; do not speak through a companion or service provider.

Offer to Shake Hands When Introduced
Always use the same good manners in interacting with a person who has a psychiatric disability that you would use in meeting any other person. Shaking hands is a uniformly acceptable and recognized signal of friendliness in American culture. A lack of simple courtesy is unacceptable to most people and tends to make everyone uncomfortable.

Make Eye Contact and Be Aware of Body Language
Like others, people with mental illness sense your discomfort. Look people in the eye when speaking to them. Maintain a relaxed posture.

Listen Attentively
If a person has difficulty in speaking or speaks in a manner that is difficult for you to understand, listen carefully—then wait for them to finish speaking. If needed, clarify what they have said. Ask short questions that can be answered by a "yes" or a "no" or by nodding the head. Never pretend to understand. Reflect what you have heard, and let the person respond.

Treat Adults as Adults
Always use common courtesy. Do not assume familiarity by using the person's first name or by touching their shoulder or arm, unless you know the person well enough to do so. Do not patronize, condescend, or threaten. Do not make decisions for the person or assume their preferences.

Do Not Give Unsolicited Advice or Assistance
If you offer any kind of assistance, wait until the offer is accepted. Then listen to the person's response and/or ask for suggestions or instructions. Do not panic or summon an ambulance or the police if a person appears to be experiencing a mental health crisis. Calmly ask the person how you can help.

Do Not Blame the Person
A person who has a mental illness has a complex, biomedical condition that is sometimes difficult to control, even with proper treatment. A person who is experiencing a mental illness cannot "just shape up" or "pull himself up by the bootstraps." It is rude, insensitive, and ineffective to tell or expect the person to do so.

Table 9.4 (continued)

Question the Accuracy of the Media Stereotypes of Mental Illness   The movies and the media have sensationalized mental illness. In reality, despite the overabundance of "psychotic killers" portrayed in movies and television, studies have shown that people with mental illness are far more likely to be victims of crime than to victimize others. Most people with mental illness never experience symptoms which include violent behavior. As with the general public, about 1–5% of all people with mental illness are exceptionally easily provoked to violence (National Alliance for the Mentally Ill 1990)
Relax!   The most important thing to remember in interacting with people who have mental health disabilities is to BE YOURSELF. Do not be embarrassed if you happen to use common expressions that seem to relate to a mental health disability, such as "I'm CRAZY about him" or "This job is driving me NUTS." ASK the person how he feels about what you have said. Chances are, you get a flippant remark and a laugh in answer.
See the Person   Beneath all the symptoms and behaviors someone with a mental illness may exhibit is a PERSON who has many of the same wants, needs, dreams, and desires as anyone else. Don't avoid people with mental health disabilities. If you are fearful or uncomfortable, learn more about mental illness. Kindness, courtesy, and patience usually smooth interactions with all kinds of people, including people who have a mental health disability.

Adapted by Mary Lee Stocks, MSW, LISW, from the Ten Commandments of Communicating with People with Disabilities, originally developed by the National Center for Access Unlimited/Chicago and United Cerebral Palsy Associations/Washington, D.C.; and a video and script developed by Irene M. Ward & Associates/Columbus, Ohio, partially supported through Ohio Development Disabilities Planning Council Grant #92-13 (1993)

9.5 Hearing and Vision Impairment

We are here dealing with the problems of mentally impaired children, but other types of disabilities, that make the communication difficult, exist. Although the health professionals participating in a study [47] reported successess in communicating effectively with patients with hearing or vision loss, many gaps remain, and instances still are present where physicians' preferences clash with patients' wishes. Examples include physicians' preferences for remote/online sign language interpreters, despite patients desire in-person interpreters. Few educational materials are available in braille, and electronic medical records may not allow documents to be printed in large font for persons with impaired vision [47].

References

1. Hepper PG. Fetal memory: does it exist? What does it do? Acta Paediatr Suppl. 1996;416:16–20. https://doi.org/10.1111/j.1651-2227.1996.tb14272.x.
2. Chorna O, Filippa M, De Almeida JS, Lordier L, Monaci MG, Hüppi P, Grandjean D, Guzzetta A. Neuroprocessing mechanisms of music during fetal and neonatal development: a role in neuroplasticity and neurodevelopment. Neural Plast. 2019;2019:3972918. https://doi.org/10.1155/2019/3972918.

3. Johnston CC, Filion F, Nuyt AM. Recorded maternal voice for preterm neonates undergoing heel lance. Adv Neonatal Care. 2007;7(5):258–66.
4. Rand K, Lahav A. Maternal sounds elicit lower heart rate in preterm newborns in the first month of life. Early Hum Dev. 2014;90(10):679–83. https://doi.org/10.1016/j.earlhum.
5. Reissland N, Mason C, Schaal B, Lincoln K. Prenatal mouth movements: can we identify co-ordinated fetal mouth and LIP actions necessary for feeding? Int J Pediatr. 2012;2012:848596. https://doi.org/10.1155/2012/848596. Epub 2012 Jul 2.
6. De Cosmi V, Scaglioni S, Agostoni C. Early taste experiences and later food choices. Nutrients. 2017;9(2):107. https://doi.org/10.3390/nu9020107.
7. Sonne J, Reddy V, Lopez-Ojeda W. Neuroanatomy, Cranial Nerve 0 (Terminal Nerve). In: StatPearls [Internet]. Treasure Island, FL: StatPearls Publishing; 2021.
8. Nagy E, Thompson P, Mayor L, Doughty H. Do foetuses communicate? Foetal responses to interactive versus non-interactive maternal voice and touch: an exploratory analysis. Infant Behav Dev. 2021;63:101562. https://doi.org/10.1016/j.infbeh.2021.101562. Epub 2021 Apr 5.
9. Anand KJ, Clancy B. Fetal pain? Pain: clinical updates. 2006;14(2).
10. Padilla N, Lagercrantz H. Making of the mind. Acta Paediatr. 2020;109(5):883–92. https://doi.org/10.1111/apa.15167. Epub 2020 Jan 31.
11. Als H, Gilkerson (1997) The role of relationship-based developmentally supportive newborn intensive care in strengthening outcome of preterm infants. Semin Perinatol 21:178–189.
12. Als H, McAnulty GB. The Newborn Individualized Developmental Care and Assessment Program (NIDCAP) with Kangaroo Mother Care (KMC): comprehensive care for preterm infants. Curr Womens Health Rev. 2011;7(3):288–301. https://doi.org/10.2174/157340411796355216.
13. Bellieni CV, et al. Alone no more: pain in premature children. Ethics and Medicine. 2003;19(1):5–10.
14. Bellieni CV, Bagnoli F, Perrone S, Nenci A, Cordelli DM, Fusi M, Ceccarelli S, Buonocore G. Effect of multisensory stimulation on analgesia in term neonates: a randomized controlled trial. Pediatr Res. 2002;51(4):460–3. https://doi.org/10.1203/00006450-200204000-00010.
15. LaGasse LL, Neal AR, Lester BM. Assessment of infant cry: acoustic cry analysis and parental perception. Ment Retard Dev Disabil Res Rev. 2005;11(1):83–93. https://doi.org/10.1002/mrdd.20050.
16. Bellieni CV, Sisto R, Cordelli DM, Buonocore G. Cry features reflect pain intensity in term newborns: an alarm threshold. Pediatr Res. 2004;55(1):142–6. https://doi.org/10.1203/01.PDR.0000099793.99608.CB. Epub 2003 Nov 6.
17. Clarici A, Travan L, Accardo A, De Vonderweid U, Bava A. Crying of a newborn child: alarm signal or protocommunication? Percept Mot Skills. 2002;95(3 Pt 1):752–4. https://doi.org/10.2466/pms.2002.95.3.752.
18. Bellieni C: Meaning and importance of weeping. New Ideas in Psychology 2017;47:72–76.
19. Sussman F. More Than Words. Courses.washington.edu. The Hanen Centre; 2012:424.
20. Mohan M, Bajaj G, Deshpande A, Anakkathil Anil M, Bhat JS. Child, parent, and play—an insight into these dimensions among children with and without receptive expressive language disorder using video-based analysis. Psychol Res Behav Manag. 2021;14:971–85. https://doi.org/10.2147/PRBM.S306733.
21. Cochet H, Byrne RW. Communication in the second and third year of life: relationships between nonverbal social skills and language. Infant Behav Dev. 2016;44:189–98. https://doi.org/10.1016/j.infbeh.2016.07.
22. Harbison AL, McDaniel J, Yoder PJ. The association of imperative and declarative intentional communication with language in young children with autism spectrum disorder: a meta-analysis. In: Research in autism spectrum disorders. Vol. 36. Elsevier; 2017:21–34.
23. Camaioni L, Perucchini P, Bellagamba F, Colonnesi C. The role of declarative pointing in developing a theory of mind. Infancy. 2004;5(3):291–308. https://doi.org/10.1207/s15327078in0503_3.
24. Bruner J. Play, thought, and language. Peabody J Educ. 1983;60(3):60–9. https://doi.org/10.1080/01619568309538407.

25. Dunham P, Dunham F. Optimal social structures and adaptive infant development; 1995. https://psycnet.apa.org/record/1995-97586-007. Accessed 23 June 2021.
26. Mirenda PL, Donnellan AM, Yoder DE. Gaze behavior: a new look at an old problem. J Autism Dev Disord. 1983;13(4):397–409. https://doi.org/10.1007/BF01531588.
27. Beukelman DR, Light J. Augmentative & alternative communication: supporting children and adults with complex communication needs. 5th ed. Baltimore, MD: Paul H. Brookes Publishing Co; 2020.
28. Rangel-Rodríguez GA, Martín MB, Blanch S, Wilkinson KM. The early development of emotional competence profile: a means to share information about emotional status and expression by children with complex communication needs. Am J Speech Lang Pathol. 2021;30(2):551–65.
29. Wilkinson KM, Na JY, Rangel-Rodríguez GA, Sowers DJ. Fostering communication about emotions: aided augmentative and alternative communication challenges and solutions. In: Ogletree BT, editor. Augmentative and alternative communication: challenges and solutions. Plural Publishing Inc; 2021. p. 313–38.
30. Reed CL, Moody EJ, Mgrublian K, Assaad S, Schey A, McIntosh DN. Body matters in emotion: restricted body movement and posture affect expression and recognition of status-related emotions. Front Psychol. 2020;11:1961.
31. Avagyan A, Mkrtchyan H, Shafa FA, Mathew JA, Petrosyan T. Effectiveness and determinant variables of augmentative and alternative communication interventions in cerebral palsy patients with communication deficit: a systematic review. Codas. 2021;33(5):e20200244. https://doi.org/10.1590/2317-1782/20202020244.
32. Light J, McNaughton D. Supporting the communication, language, and literacy development of children with complex communication needs: state of the science and future research priorities. Assist Technol. 2011;24(1):34–44.
33. Al-Yahyai ANS, Arulappan J, Matua GA, Al-Ghafri SM, Al-Sarakhi SH, Al-Rahbi KKS, Jayapal SK. Communicating to non-speaking critically ill patients: augmentative and alternative communication technique as an essential strategy. SAGE Open Nurs. 2021;7:23779608211015234. https://doi.org/10.1177/23779608211015234.
34. Barker RM, Romski M, Sevcik RA, Adamson LB, Smith AL, Bakeman R. Intervention focus moderates the association between initial receptive language and language outcomes for toddlers with developmental delay. Augment Altern Commun. 2019;35(4):263–73. https://doi.org/10.1080/07434618.2019.1686770. Epub 2019 Dec 23
35. Infingardi Kruger S, Berberian AP, et al. Delimitation of the area named augmentative and alternative communication (AAC). Rev CEFAC. 2017;19(2):265–76.
36. Griffiths T, Bloch S, Price K, Clarke M. Alternative and augmentative communication. In: Cowan D, Najafi L, editors. Handbook of electronic assistive technology. Academic Press, 2019. p. 181–213.
37. Holyfield C. Comparative effects of picture symbol with paired text and text-only augmentative and alternative communication representations on communication from children with autism spectrum disorder. Am J Speech Lang Pathol. 2021;30(2):584–97. https://doi.org/10.1044/2020_AJSLP-20-00099. Epub 2021 Feb 8.
38. Alzrayer NM. Transitioning from a low- to high-tech Augmentative and Alternative Communication (AAC) system: effects on augmented and vocal requesting. Augment Altern Commun. 2020;36(3):155–65. https://doi.org/10.1080/07434618.2020.1813196. Epub 2020 Oct 5
39. Ivy S, Robbins A, Kerr MG. Adapted picture exchange communication system using tangible symbols for young learners with significant multiple disabilities. Augment Altern Commun. 2020;36(3):166–78. https://doi.org/10.1080/07434618.2020.1826051. Epub 2020 Oct 7.
40. Broomfield K, Craig C, Smith S, Jones G, Judge S, Sage K. Creativity in public involvement: supporting authentic collaboration and inclusive research with seldom heard voices. Res Involv Engagem. 2021;7(1):17. https://doi.org/10.1186/s40900-021-00260-7.
41. Creer S, Enderby P, Judge S, John A. Prevalence of people who could benefit from augmentative and alternative communication (AAC) in the UK: determining the need. Int J Lang

Commun Disord. 2016;51(6):639–53. https://doi.org/10.1111/1460-6984.12235. Epub 2016 Apr 26.
42. Foley DC, McCutcheon H. Detecting pain in people with an intellectual disability. Accid Emerg Nurs. 2004;12(4):196–200. https://doi.org/10.1016/j.aaen.2004.06.002.
43. Breau LM, Finley GA, McGrath PJ, Camfield CS. Validation of the non-communicating children's pain checklist-postoperative version. Anesthesiology. 2002;96(3):528–35. https://doi.org/10.1097/00000542-200203000-00004. Erratum in: Anesthesiology 2002 Sep;97(3):769.
44. Massaro M, Ronfani L, Ferrara G, Badina L, Giorgi R, D'Osualdo F, Taddio A, Barbi E. A comparison of three scales for measuring pain in children with cognitive impairment. Acta Paediatr. 2014;103(11):e495–500. https://doi.org/10.1111/apa.12748. Epub 2014 Aug 15.
45. McGuire BE, Kennedy S. Pain in people with an intellectual disability. Curr Opin Psychiatry. 2013;26(3):270–5. https://doi.org/10.1097/YCO.0b013e32835fd74c.
46. Ilievski V, Coneva A. Communication of persons with mental disorders. jAHR. 2013;4(7):377–84.
47. Agaronnik N, Campbell EG, Ressalam J, Iezzoni LI. Communicating with patients with disability: perspectives of practicing physicians. J Gen Intern Med. 2019;34(7):1139–45. https://doi.org/10.1007/s11606-019-04911-0. Epub 2019 Mar 18.
48. Messeri A, Atzori B, Vagnoli L. Interactive media versus human activities to reduce waiting room anxiety: what is the best option for children with disabilities? Dev Med Child Neurol. 2018;60(6):539.
49. Scrooby B, Roos SD, Gmeiner AC. Fasiliterende kommunikasie met die verstandelik vertraagde persoon tydens die behandeling van geringe ongesteldhede [Effective communication with the mentally challenged person during treatment of minor ailments]. Curationis. 2000;23(3):93–103. Afrikaans.
50. San Diego State University. Tips for interacting with people with mental health disabilities. 2021. https://newscenter.sdsu.edu/student_affairs/sds/tip-mental-health.aspx

Part IV
What Is a Good Behavior (Aka Ethics)

Palliative care has several features that are commonly highlighted as an "ethical" pull. It is the case of end-of-life decisions, correct patient–doctor relationship, and the huge field of the rights of the child. Therefore, we cannot treat this topic without dealing with bioethics. The problem is that everyone is sure of what "being ethical" means, but, if asked, few will give a proper answer. Here, we will deal with ethics, to get ethics away from improvization, giving an overall insight of this branch of philosophy. You will discover ideas and situations you did not imagine before. Then, we will see how ethics concerns the minor, paradoxically discovering that even the minor has ethical parameters to follow. We will deal with the problem of informed consent, parental potesty, and end-of-life decisions. Finally, we will analyze if, when we are dealing with a minor, we have to maintain the same ethical standards that we use with an adult.

Dear reader before approaching the new section of the book, please take a moment for yourself, sit back and let that sink in…

Intermezzo

Protocols and the False Reassurance

"I have been very lucky in recent years, luck has spoiled me, I had been restless, but restlessness without luck leads to nothing. What I would have to do now first would be properly a check to the den to accurately verify its defense and all the imaginable eventualities in relation to it, the elaboration of a defense plan and the related construction project and then, immediately at work, fresh as a young man. The necessary work for which—incidentally said—It is obviously too late, but it would be the necessary work, is the excavation of some large exploratory tunnel which properly only has the consequence of leaving me without defense and despite all my strength exposed to danger, in the mad fear that he may appear too soon. (…) In reality there is no peace here either. Danger is lurking as before."

Franz Kafka—The Den

Are You Sure to Know What "Ethics" Really Is?

10

10.1 Ethics, Virtues, and Protocols

10.1.1 First Premise: The Nonsensical Adjective "Ethical"

A problem with ethics is that we use the word "ethical" as an adjective for the word "conduct," to say "a good conduct." But the expression "ethical conduct" is a tautology, a meaningless repetition of words (such as "burning heat" or "spoken word"), as if we were saying "conduct of conduct." In fact, the word "ethics" comes from the Greek term "ethos," which means "way of acting," behavior, conduct. The word ethics has lost its original sense: the adjective "ethical" did not mean "good," but originally means "behavioral," and is an attribute of the word "virtue."

To understand this, we should point out that Aristotle divided virtues into ethical virtues (those about human behavior, such as justice) and dianoetic virtues (those about human thinking, such as wisdom) [1]; he dealt with that in his book Ethics to Nicomachus, a book about the behavior he suggests to his son Nicomachus. So, for a good life, he used to suggest the virtues of behavior and the virtues of thinking. For him, the point was not being ethical (which etymologically is a nonsense), but being virtuous [2]. Thus, what we now call ethical should be called virtuous.

Then the question arises: what is a virtue? And the answer comes from its etymology "vir," which means "man" (or rather "human," but we should be indulgent with the male-centered ancient philosophers): virtue is what makes the man (human being) a Man (a Human); and what does it make the human being a Human Being? For millennia, this has been self-explanatory: to be honest, responsible, and so forth. With the time, virtues have been replaced by principles; but without virtues, principles are a form of alienation, the distance for humans from being Human. All the principles (beneficence, non-maleficence, justice, and autonomy) are to be considered for what they are: signs to facilitate the path of the virtues; unfortunately, now ethics seems just a matter of principles to respect. Gunther Anders [3, 4] wrote

© The Author(s), under exclusive license to Springer Nature Switzerland AG 2022
C. V. Bellieni, *A New Holistic-Evolutive Approach to Pediatric Palliative Care*,
https://doi.org/10.1007/978-3-030-96256-2_10

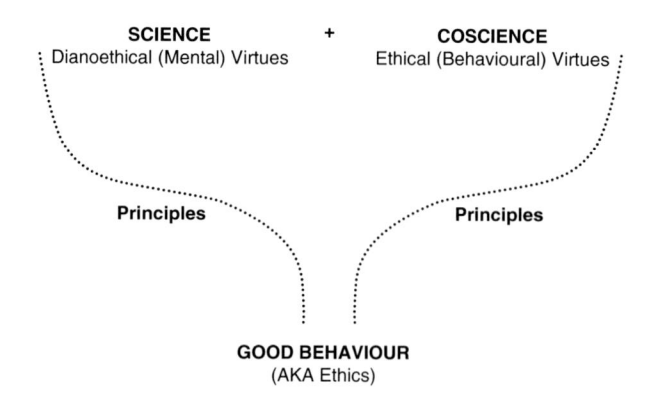

```
            SCIENCE            +           COSCIENCE
    Dianoethical (Mental) Virtues      Ethical (Behavioural) Virtues


            Principles                       Principles


                         GOOD BEHAVIOUR
                           (AKA Ethics)
```

Fig. 10.1 Relationship among virtues, principles, and ethics. Without virtues no behavior can be said good, or ethical. The so-called ethical principle are just the boundaries of the virtues; principles are another way of saying that virtues should be applied "with measure" (in Greek "kata metròn"). Science and conscience are the bases of the good medical behavior, and here we notice that the word medical is derived from "metròn" which is the corollary of the two above areas of science and conscience (see text)

beautiful pages on this topic: he explained that humans want to replace their responsibilities with protocols and principles, because they have a sort of envy of the stillness and lack of responsibilities of the machines: he used to call it, the "Promethean envy."

This is the matter, and it would be sufficient to understand what really is needed for a good behavior: following and cultivating our inner virtues (Fig. 10.1).

Unfortunately, this is an old story, and ethics as well as bioethics have become complicated as far as they have abandoned this simple source.

Therefore, in the rest of this book, to avoid misunderstanding, we use the word "ethical" not in its pure sense we have just explained, but as it is commonly used: a synonym of "good" referred to our behavior.

10.1.2 Second Premise: Mixing Up Ethics with Rules

Treating a patient is never a mechanical act: it implies our active responsibility. There are three main ways to misunderstand what an ethical behavior is: (1) just following the law code, (2) just following what we instinctively approve, (3) doing what is the current fashion. All good intentions, sure; but they also are a reduction of ethics to norms, to instinct, or to conformism. In no case, these ways of acting imply our active responsibility. Ethics implies our personal choice and our personal adherence to inner virtues, rather than being a setting of rules; it implies the use of our reason and of our sensibility. Nonetheless, in Western countries the dichotomies of true and false, good and bad, fair and unfair, have disappeared in the common speech; to approve a behavior, we do not say "it is good," but "it is correct," "it is consequential" because the moral virtues and categories (good, bad, wrong) are now considered obsolete.

Two are the most diffuse strategies of common ethics, namely utilitarianism [5], and principlism [6]. Utilitarianism invites to weight the effects of an action and allows to do it if the pros outweights the cons. Principlism gives a series of principles and allows an action if these principles are respected [7]. Both seem easy tools and are useful to the clinician. They are fine standpoints to be introduced into the arena of our behavior. But they risk to confuse the good behavior and the good attitudes with a cold series of rules, or a balance between different outcomes, and nothing more. While ethics is something more indeed.

10.2 A Synoptic Vision

An ethical behavior cannot follow mere principles; otherwise, it becomes cold and repulsive; nor can it be the copy of stereotyped behaviors, such as that of computers, of the herd of animals, or of the mechanisms of a gear. Ethical behavior must follow virtues, which are innate to the person, certainly with different shades over the centuries and traditions, but perennial in their basic structure. The reason is easy to understand: a good behavior is a human behavior, has the features of human freedom, of realism, rationality, and empathy; otherwise, it builds walls between the people, instead of making bridges of shared choices. For a choice to be shared, principles are important, and mere weighting the outcomes is correct, but the human factor is determinant, and a good behavior is obtained considering principles not as supreme courts, but as embankments of a flow of the human behavior that has chosen to be virtuous.

Therefore, in the foreword of this book we talked about a culture of the synopsis, namely of "watching together." It has two meanings.

The first is "watching the whole scenario": it is the holistic view of the nature of the problem. Modern medicine does not limit its field to treating symptoms or overcoming disease; but it is a medicine that is close to the person, to their surroundings, grafted into their tribe, their ethnic group, their geographical area, their family and mindset. It is a medicine that looks at the symptoms, but also at the surroundings social degradation, the story of the patients, and that respects their mood and style. This means having an overall view, a bird's eye view of the problem, as if we were preparing a battle, and would arrange the field, the cannons, the armies, the time, and the resources.

The second step is "watching along with the patient." We cannot think of a medical treatment that deserves the term "ethical" if not by standing together with the patient. Searching proximity, living together, touching, measuring, and shielding the patient. It is in daily life that the doctor's ability to be a Doctor emerges. People are wary of strangers, yet how many times in hospitals they are in the hands of someone they do not know! Watching together means that there is not only a contract between us, but a path that we have started together and that we will continue after the end of the disease, though sometimes only in our memory.

In pediatric palliative care, all this has a very evident practical implication, which we summarize in three points:

- Encouraging the presence of the doctor who knows the child and the family, so as not to traumatize them with strangers: all the other medical figures will be "consultants".
- Looking, talking, visiting, getting to know the patients, and revisiting them again is imperative for every health professional. Spending time to know the patient with familiarity and acquaintance means understanding those things that the patient cannot express in words.
- Cooperating affably with the other doctors who treat the child. This will be useful for the whole process, but above all it will give the patient and his family a sense of security.

10.3 Our Ethical Responsibilities

We can harm someone with either active or permissive behaviors [8]. It is self-evident that killing the innocent is a non-ethical behavior [9], but it is also unethical to permit harming the innocent by allowing others to do it, by decreasing our level of alertness [10]. Thus, paraphrasing what Plato wrote about knowledge (fourth century BC, see [11]), a behavior is unethical (it is not able to perfectly know and therefore to adapt its virtues to its object) not necessarily when it is perverse, but even when it is a mechanical imitation of the virtues (that for Plato were part of the metaphysical "world of the ideas"), behaving by routine and not by conviction. We can behave in a virtuous way or in a virtual way; the latter is when we pretend a good attitude just applying rules and not showing a sincere interest for the patient, being fake, being an imitation, an alteration of the original virtue [12]; and imitations of virtues are no more virtues because even a robot can do them. To exercise the virtues, you need your humanity, inspiration, originality, genius; an imitation is a scam.

An imitation of a virtue is better than no virtue, but not much better. Plato [13] used to talk of arts as copy of the nature, and as nature as a copy of the world of the ideas. This series of copies provoked a sort of degeneration from the original. Similarly, we can affirm that the further one moves away from the original human behavior, the more the thing or the action becomes bad because the source is lost. When one moves away from the Human, the behavior is unethical. There are three ways to behave as a copy of a Human:

- Acting like a robot with stereotyped repetitive actions.
- Imitating a computer, perfect in execution, but without making anything beyond what is prescribed.
- Imitating animals by letting the reasoning of the herd prevail over that of the individual.

10.3 Our Ethical Responsibilities

Ultimately, an action ceases to be virtuous when it is a bad copy of the human, an impure, imperfect, though sophisticated copy [10].

For example:

1. When a man screws a bolt repeatedly, it is not an original action, but a copy of a copy: it is the copy of a machine that screws the bolt. If I give bad news to the patient by ideally following a manual, I am a copy of how a robot would do it.
2. A person who performs delicate activities, following only and exclusively what is written in protocols, makes a copy of what a computer would do, which in turn copies man; they behave "like a person," but not "as a person," because no protocol can describe everything, protocols do not indicate the exceptions, and therefore you cannot find empathy, modesty, sensitivity in their actions. For example, if someone gives you sad news on your health by simply following a protocol (and many protocols exist describing point-by-point how to give bad news), you will perceive a flaw in their humanity, you will feel your humanity is not being respected but mocked: they have behaved as if they were computers.
3. Finally, whoever follows the majority, whatever it says, is like an animal that follows the herd, the flock, they are like a sheep. It is what was being "unauthentic" for Martin Heidegger, following the "gerede" ("idle conversation," in German) or the conventions of the majority. If the majority of people think that disability can make a person's life unworthy, or if they think that pain should be gone through in silence, or any other idea, and you follow as a routine these theses of the flock, you are just one in the flock.

Knowledge of the object is the prerequisite of good behavior; Marcuse in 1964 wrote: "Ethics is epistemology and epistemology is ethics" [14]. The term "epistemology" derives from the greek word "episteme" that means "knowledge". This means that for a good behavior the first step is not following rules nor imitating, but becoming aware, according to rationality, realism, and empathy, as we will see later. In fact, the spirit of knowledge is, according to Aristotle, the correspondence between our attitude and the essence of a thing, summarized by the expression "adjustment of the thing and of the intellect" (in Latin: "adaequatio rei et intellectus"). This expression means that our empathy and virtues should be active, and that, simultaneously, the object of our observation should be made visible, acknowledgeable [15]. Thus, three conditions are necessary to this end: reasonableness, realism, and empathy [16].

- Reasonableness: to approach reality trying not to censor anything [17], embracing it according to all its factors, but at the same time without forgetting anything about us: our history and our desires.
- Realism: it means that the method of approaching an issue or a person is determined by the person or the subject [18]; and that we are willing to change any opinion that we have preformed if the reality imposes it.
- Empathy: the reality really interests us: without interest, all ethical judgment is formal and superficial, and therefore artificial [19].

10.4 Children's Ethical Responsibilities

Talking of children's ethical responsibility is a paradox, of course. Here we outline it, not with the aim of saying how *they* should behave, but what *we* should expect from their behavior. The conclusion of this paragraph is that children behave ethically when they behave like children, namely when they decide with their instinct guided by the love for their parents, not by full rationality, that they are developing bit by bit. So, let's learn what to expect from them.

Does the child have no ethical responsibilities? Of course, they have some, although in a different way than adults [20]. What is the ethical responsibility of a subject who does not have the rational capacity to distinguish *what* is good from *what* is evil? It is their affective responsibility of distinguishing *who* is good from *who* is evil unto them. This is their affective responsibility, a word derived from the Latin verb "afficio", which means "being close to somebody" [21]. Thus, an ethical responsibility (paradoxically but at least etimologically) exists for the minor. The difference between adults' and minors' ethics is that the former concerns volition, the latter regards instinct. Nonetheless, even if instincual, this responsibility exists in children; it will become more voluntary as the child grows up. It is easier to understand this, if we consider that the word responsibility comes from the Latin verb respondeo, which means "to fulfill a promise," not in the sense of a voluntaristic commitment, but honestly watching and being stuck to someone. For instance, the "Observational Learning Approach" [22], developed more than a half century ago by Albert Bandura, suggests that it is possible to promote honesty in children by allowing them to observe a peer's display of honest behavior [23]. This is how virtues are learned.

This should be clear: ethics for children is solely behaving accordingly to their age, and their age's law is the progressive capability of following an encounter, of being affectively stuck with their loved ones. As time goes by, the responsibility of behaving accordingly to their age and of distinguishing evil from good people, acquires more and more conscious and free attachment to the people who are taking care of them, along with their capacity of response, and with their sense of responsibility. Being moral for a child is not following rules, having fear of punishments or having senses of guilt that curb their inner impulses. It is just behaving according to their age, according to what their affective sight permits, becoming social, being attached to the reality and the people who form their reality.

This is their affective responsibility [24]: responding to an affective solicitation. It is learned since the first years of life and is the moral and existential basis of every social being, including the child. If it is not learned, children lose coherence with themselves and with their parents. Also the word coherence, as well as the word responsibility, means to be stuck to something (from the latin verb "haereo"). In the earliest stages of life, one learns to be human simply through their coherence with those who are the roots of their vital organism. Being coherent is the way for the minor to be responsible, hence ethical. In sum, children's responsibilty is not to distinguish abstractly between "good and evil", but between "good and evil people" and follow the former; it is intrinsecal to their behaving since birth, as the attachment is not an acquired behavior but an innate one. This is the law of the baby, who instinctively stucks to their mother since birth.

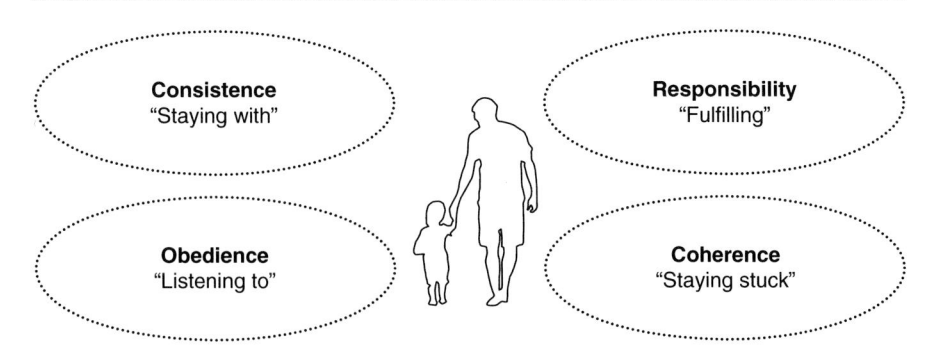

Fig. 10.2 The real meanings of the words that describe children's behavior, that here we call "ethical" duties

Children thrive by osmosis [25, 26], by imitation of what is in front of them, mirroring the movements, the sounds, the steps of their parents, watching what happens, who is good or evil unto them, noble maybe in the Socratic-maieutic way [27].

Listening (not necessarily obeying but also not ignoring) to whom is in front of us is the law of life, from the cradle to the grave. And in Latin listening to whom we have in front of us is said with a verb obtained by joining the prefix "ob" (in front of) and the verb audire (to hear): oboedire in Latin and in English to obey. Thus, to obey is not a synonym of "doing something for the fear of ominous consequences": it simply means "to listen to what is evident," to the reality in front of us (despite the mere negative sense this word usually has) [28]. Like the words coherence and responsibility, also "to obey" pivots on the concept of "being close" to those we reckon worth respecting and loving. In this sense, and only in this, obedience is an ethical duty of the child (Fig. 10.2).

This shows an important concept for our palliative care work. We have said that an act is unethical when it is a copy; therefore, the child is not ethical when they pretend to have an autonomy that is not typical of their age. You cannot ask children to decide on a treatment, but you can ask them if they can tolerate it, and to trust in what their caregivers are proposing to them. This imposes to the parents to behave without authoritanianism and laxity, and to the baby to behave watching to whom they know are worth of trust. This dialectic behavior is the base of palliative care.

In conclusion, allegiance is not an imperative for the children; it is the way they thrive.

References

1. Sachs J. Aristotle Nicomachean ethics: translation, glossary and introductory essay. Focus Publishing; 2002.
2. Begley AM. Facilitating the development of moral insight in practice: teaching ethics and teaching virtue. Nurs Philos. 2006;7(4):257–65. https://doi.org/10.1111/j.1466-769X.2006.00284.x.
3. Anders G. Die Antiquiertheit des Menschen 1: Über die Seele im Zeitalter der zweiten industriellen Revolution. München: C.H. Beck; 1956.
4. Anders G. On Promethean Shame. In: Müller C, editor. Prometheanism: technology, digital culture and human obsolescence. Rowman and Litlefield; 2016. p. 29–95.

5. Scarre G. Utilitarianism. Routledge; 1° edizione (7 ottobre); 1995.
6. Beauchamp TL, Rautlich O. Principlism. In: ten Have T, editor. Encyclopedia of global bioethics. Springer; 2016.
7. Sorell T. The limits of principlism and recourse to theory: the example of telecare. Ethic Theory Moral Prac. 2011;14:369–82.
8. Gostin LO, Gostin KG. A broader liberty: J.S. Mill, paternalism and the public's health. Public Health. 2009;123(3):214–21. https://doi.org/10.1016/j.puhe.2008.12.024. Epub 2009 Feb 27.
9. Quong J. Killing in self-defense. Ethics. 2009;119(3):507–37.
10. Arendt H. Eichmann in Jerusalem. A report on the Banality of Evil. Penguin Classics; 2006.
11. Plato. Phaedrus. Digireads.com Publishing; 2016.
12. Tate J. Plato and the "Imitation". Class Q. 1932;26(3-4):161–9.
13. Plato. The Republic. 3rd ed. Penguin; 2007.
14. Marcuse H. The unidimensional man. Beacon Press; 1964.
15. Prior AN. Correspondence theory of truth. In: Encyclopedia of philosophy, vol. 2. Macmillan; 1969. p. 223–4.
16. Bellieni CV. Padroni della vita? Piccolo vademecum di bioetica. Florence, Italy: SEF Ed; 2006.
17. Rescher N. Reasonableness in ethics. Philos Stud. 1954;5:58–62.
18. Werner R. Ethical realism. Ethics. 1983;93(4:653–79.
19. Slote M. The ethics of care and empathy. Routledge Ed. 2007;
20. UNICEF. Children's rights and responsibilities. 2009. https://www.unicef.org/uganda/media/5591/file/UGDA%20CRC%20child%20friendly%20booklet%20final.pdf
21. Hall DMB. Children's rights and responsibilities. Arch Dis Child. 2005;90:171–3.
22. Ma F, Heyman GD, Jing C, Fu Y, Compton BJ, Xu F, Lee K. Promoting honesty in young children through observational learning. J Exp Child Psychol. 2018;167:234–45. https://doi.org/10.1016/j.jecp.2017.11.003. Epub 2017 Nov 28.
23. Bandura A, Grusec JE, Menlove FL. Observational learning as a function of symbolization and incentive set. Child Dev. 1966;37(3):499–506.
24. Feltz A, Cova F. Moral responsibility and free will: a meta-analysis. Conscious Cogn. 2014;30:234–46. https://doi.org/10.1016/j.concog.2014.08.012. Epub 2014 Oct 13.
25. Snow CE. Mothers' speech to children learning language. Child Dev. 1972;43(2):549–65.
26. Užgiris I, Broome S, Kruper JC. Imitation in mother-child conversations: a focus on the mother. In: Speidel GE, Nelson KE, editors. The many faces of imitation in language learning. Springer series in language and communication, vol. 24. New York, NY: Springer; 2011. https://doi.org/10.1007/978-1-4612-1011-5_5.
27. Rousseau JJ. Emile. Or on education. Basic Books Ed; 1979.
28. Carlsmith JM, Lepper MR, Landauer TK. Children's obedience to adult requests: interactive effects of anxiety arousal and apparent punitiveness of the adult. J Pers Soc Psychol. 1974;30(6):822–8. https://doi.org/10.1037/h0037530.

The Limits of Parental Authority

11.1 Parents Applying Ethical Rules

Pediatric ethics also addresses another specific point: how can a parent take decisions for the child? Here, I emphasize how the three guidelines of ethics I mentioned earlier (rationality, empathy, and realism) find their application.

- *Rationality.* Parents have to use rationality, that is they should consider all the factors involved to take children's health-related decisions. These are some questions they would consider. "Is the child feeling pain?" "Can they bear it?" "Is the treatment too expensive?" "Does the child interact with the doctors?" "Are doctors suggesting to continuing treatments?" "Does the environment affect the child's response to therapy?" "Are children too lonely?" "Are they accompanied in these days of fatigue?" "Can they express their opinion?"
- *Realism.* Parents will also have to use realism, namely being able to change their minds if the reality urges them to do it. "Has the pain level changed?" "Has the child's level of acceptance of treatments changed?" "Has the prognosis changed?" "Has an external event occurred, by which the child could change his attitude (e.g., the death of a relative, the birth of a brother, or a visit of a friend)?"
- *Empathy.* Finally, parents will use the empathy, that is thinking that their child's interest does not always coincide with their own; in fact, sometimes the sick child is not terminal, while their parents are exhausted and overwhelmed; or the child can expressly say that they can no longer bear an intensive and invasive care, while their parents do not want to give up.

Parents should take decisions on behalf of the child; but can parental acceptance or rejection of a treatment be an absolute court? Can parents decide for the baby the same way they would decide for themselves, that is, without barriers of any kind? If the adult patient rejects a therapy, doctors can disagree, but the patients are the supreme judges of their own health. Instead, in the case of children, parents can only act in the interests of the child when dealing with accepting or withdrawing therapies [1]. According to some legislatures, parents can decide to suspend the care exclusively in the interest of the "health and life" of the minor [2]. This distinction should be clear: parents are not the owners of the child and cannot make any decision on their behalf if it is not explicitly in the minor's interest. This reminds what commonly laws impose to people in the case of decisions in the economic sphere: a parent cannot sell without a good reason the goods that for some reason already belong to the offspring, while they could sell (even unreasonably) what is their own. Therefore, the consent or request of the parents for the interruption of vital treatments can only take place if it is in the best interest of the minor. We will see what the limits of the "best interest" criterion are, and when the suspension of treatments is really worth for the child.

Can parents decide to withdraw life-saving treatments because a future severe disability is predicted? The prognosis of a severe disability shows a future life without autonomy, in need of continuous care, and are favorable to withdraw vital care to avoid a life with disability [3]. But there are two possible objections. The first is that sometimes the future disability is just hypothetical and not yet defined, or this disability affects only minor aspects of life, and this should be weighted to make an appropriate decision in favor of the child. The second is that the mere disability is not enough to justify end-of-life choices: only a minority of people with disabilities ask for death, showing that the equation between disability and unbearable life is not automatic, and the equation between disability and life unworthy of living is a way of stigmatizing and offending the disabled, describing them as alive by mistake [4]. In both cases, it seems that suspending life-saving treatments is not in the interest of the patient unless suffering is present or surely predictable, as we will see when we shall deal with the *pain principle*.

11.2 End-of-Life Requests

Boundaries have been fixed to limit the State interventions in the field of personal health. Every human being has an inviolable right: there can be no intervention, even by the State itself, to impose medical treatment against their will. This is stated by the Declaration of Human Rights, as well as by the Supreme Court of the United States: "No right is considered more sacred or more jealously preserved by customary law than the right of each individual to the possession and control of his own person, without coercion or interference from others" [5]. However, this is not an absolute right: the State can intervene to force someone to receive medical treatment, when something seriously endangers the patient's health or the health of others.

Sometimes the patient does not accept a treatment without showing why, and in this case—for adults—this treatment is withheld. Anyway, suspending a medical treatment without explicit reasons can pose several problems. The risk is that patients can exercise this choice under external pressure, under an altered state of mind or that they are not really aware of the decision they are making. For example, when their real desire is limited to not receiving chemotherapy or transfusions, but they ask a total withdrawal of therapies. It would be correct—in extreme cases, in which refusal to treatment entails a serious risk for the patient—that an evaluation of the real patients' knowledge of what their treatments are is made, an assessment of the psychological state of the subject is requested, and the social service or psychologist is consulted.

Several problems are raised by the requests of assisted suicide or euthanasia. This is a really critical point, and, despite several States allow a consent to this request, two reflections are appropriate.

First, freedom of choice. In several cases, the patient is so overwhelmed that they ask to die: is this a free choice? We should not mix up freedom and loneliness, but sometimes it happens; but some final choices can be overcome after a substantial change of therapies and environmental situation [6, 7]. Second, a philosophic point is worth considering. Immanuel Kant so explained the prohibition of suicide: "Suicide is found mainly among those who have alchemized the happiness of life. It is on the crest of the intrinsic and inalienable dignity of life, unlike other human goods or possessions, that the moral prohibition of suicide is based" [8]. A subordinate factor to the prohibition is the fact that suicide can be destructive to the community by inducing a sense of resignation, disgust, terror, and even emulation [9]. Moreover, the break of the Hippocratic Oath, "I will not administer to anyone, even if asked, a deadly drug, nor will I suggest such advice" [10]] is to be reminded as a threat to the basis of medical activity.

In the case of pediatric palliative care, the case for assisted suicide or euthanasia is delicate and has peculiar boundaries. The minors can refuse treatments; they can also ask to die, but their words must be correctly interpreted, for the age they have, and the poor development of their decision-making and rational faculties. Sometimes it may be wondered if a child is asking suicide in the interest of the parents (who look excessively concerned about the pain the baby is feeling, who have economic interests to guarantee, or who are deeply exhausted). An adult who asks for a child's assisted suicide or euthanasia on the behalf of the children "because they asked me to," should receive careful information about this point.

In several cases, euthanasia is requested for unbearable suffering and pain; or for having no positive perspective of a satisfying life. In a recent review, most Dutch pediatricians felt pediatric assisted death was conceivable, even under the age of 12 if requested by the parents: they seemed to be driven by a sense of duty to relieve suffering [11]. However, the pediatric palliativist is in first line to avoid this unbearable suffering [12]: euthanasia can seem a shortcut to rule off further attempts to relieve pain or a less invasive treatment. A recent statement issued by International Association for Hospice and Palliative Care (IAHPC) so reports: "In countries and states where euthanasia and/or assisted suicide are legal, IAHPC agrees that palliative care units should not be responsible for overseeing or administering these practices. The law or policies should include provisions so that any health professional who objects must be allowed to deny participating" [13].

References

1. Birchley G. The theorisation of 'best interests' in bioethical accounts of decision-making. BMC Med Ethics. 2021;22(1):68. https://doi.org/10.1186/s12910-021-00636-0.
2. Di Paolo M, Gori F, Papi M, Turillazzi E. A review and analysis of new Italian law 219/2017: 'provisions for informed consent and advance directives treatment'. BMC Med Ethics. 2019;20:17.
3. Kopelman LM. Rejecting the Baby Doe rules and defending a "negative" analysis of the Best Interests Standard. J Med Philos. 2005;30(4):331–52. https://doi.org/10.1080/03605310591008487.
4. Janvier A, Barrington KJ, Payot A. A time for hope: guidelines for the perinatal management of extremely preterm birth. Arch Dis Child Fetal Neonatal Ed. 2020;105(3):230–1. https://doi.org/10.1136/archdischild-2019-318553. Epub 2020 Mar 10.
5. Thrasher J. SELF-OWNERSHIP AS PERSONAL SOVEREIGNTY. Social Philosophy & Policy Foundation; 2019. p. 116–33.
6. Blikshavn T, Husum TL, Magelssen M. Four reasons why assisted dying should not be offered for depression. J Bioeth Inq. 2017;14(1):151–7. https://doi.org/10.1007/s11673-016-9759-4. Epub 2016 Dec 8.
7. Marcoux I, Onwuteaka-Philipsen BD, Jansen-van der Weide MC, van der Wal G. Withdrawing an explicit request for euthanasia or physician-assisted suicide: a retrospective study on the influence of mental health status and other patient characteristics. Psychol Med. 2005;35(9):1265–74. https://doi.org/10.1017/S0033291705005465.
8. Uleman J. No King and No Torture: Kant on Suicide and Law. Kantian Review. 2016;21(1):77–100.
9. Montanari Vergallo G, Gulino M, Bersani G, Rinaldi R. Euthanasia and physician-assisted suicide for patients with depression: thought-provoking remarks. Riv Psichiatr. 2020;55(2):119–28. https://doi.org/10.1708/3333.33027.
10. Singhal S. Do no harm: the Hippocratic Oath. Natl Med J India. 2019;32(6):375. https://doi.org/10.4103/0970-258X.303624.
11. Bolt EE, Flens EQ, Pasman HR, Willems D, Onwuteaka-Philipsen BD. Physician-assisted dying for children is conceivable for most Dutch paediatricians, irrespective of the patient's age or competence to decide. Acta Paediatr. 2017;106(4):668–75. https://doi.org/10.1111/apa.13620. Epub 2016 Nov 14.
12. Möller HJ. The ongoing discussion on termination of life on request. A review from a German/European perspective. Int J Psychiatry Clin Pract. 2021;25(1):2–18. https://doi.org/10.1080/13651501.2020.1797097. Epub 2020 Jul 30.
13. De Lima L, Woodruff R, Pettus K, Downing J, Buitrago R, Munyoro E, Venkateswaran C, Bhatnagar S, Radbruch L. International Association for Hospice and Palliative Care position statement: euthanasia and physician-assisted suicide. J Palliat Med. 2017;20(1):8–14. https://doi.org/10.1089/jpm.2016.0290. Epub 2016 Nov 29.

To the Depth of Health Care 12

12.1 The Words That Describe Health Care

To fully understand the aim of the daily work in palliative care units, it is mandatory to be aware of the basic words that describe health care. The words of health care have a bright origin and illuminate the way for anyone involved in this mission. They have a deep relationship with bioethics, and discovering their real meaning will be of great utility.

The words "care" and "cure" mean that someone stands close to our heart: they derive from the word "cor" that in Latin means "heart". Actually, the cure has to do with the heart, with having somebody in the heart, with the idea that taking care of someone is letting them feel enclosed in our deepest depth.

The term "medical" (hence the name "medicine") comes from the Latin "medeo" ("I measure"), which means assessing the patient's needs, their acts, signs, parameters, getting our eyes stuck to the patient, in order to understand, to weight, to measure their symptoms and signs, but also their aspirations, desires and fears.

To heal (and also the word "health") derives from a root similar to that of the adjective "whole," emphasizing the idea that the medical activity concerns not a part, but the entire person.

In languages other than English, the medical words indicate a similar interest of the medicine for the whole person and for the human relationship. "Cuidados" (the Spanish word for Care) comes from the Latin verb "Cogitatum," literally "thought," but its etymology is interesting to know, because it is "to do together" ("cum" = with and "gerere" = to do), "to be together," "to be partners." In Italian, the word "guarire" (to cure) derives from a Germanic root that means "to shield," because who cures not only defeats diseases, but also protects the person who is in his hands. In French, the word for "care" is "soin," that has a common derivation with the word "besoin" (need). In short, the art of health implies a vital sharing, closeness, compassion with the sick. Too often we hear these words used in a cold, bureaucratic and mechanical way: we hear about healing or health as mere abstract rights, or as parts of a contract. In official acts, these words are obscure and abstract.

12.2 Health: Satisfaction Socially Supported

Let's consider the word "health." The term health was defined in 1948 by the World Health Organization as a state of complete psychological, physical, and social well-being [1]. Let's reflect on it. If health is the sum of all these perfections, nobody on earth will be ever entitled to enjoy it. Because nobody will never have a complete state of perfect equilibrium [2, 3]. Of course, this definition was set to antagonize the idea that health is the mere absence of diseases; but this solution is worse than the problem. If we want to give a realistic definition of health, we should wonder when we feel not healthy. We shall not answer: "when I can do things that nobody can do," but "when I can do things that persons of my condition (age, background, environment) can do." This means that we feel healthy when we feel satisfied. Clearly, we might equivocate, feeling falsely satisfied for settling down, or for ignoring the severity of our condition; it is for this reason that satisfaction is not enough to be healthy; it should be supported by someone who can add objectivity to our perception. In other words, we can say that health is a state of "satisfaction socially supported." This also means that health is even attainable for people with diseases. An old man would feel healthy when they can do things adequate to elderly; a child is not healthy if they can teach or manage a company, but if they can run and study [4, 5]. A person with a physical disability would not feel healthy if they want to run and climb, but if they settle for what they can realistically do. In fact, the concept of satisfaction is parallel to having a satisfying quality of life [6]; and this is not precluded to people with disabilities [7, 8]. On this wake, Krahn and colleagues [9] have defined health as "the dynamic balance of physical, mental, social, and existential well-being in adapting to conditions of life and the environment." This means that the sense of well-being is relative to one's state and conditions; here, it is worth pointing out how similar is this concept of adaptation to that of satisfaction we used before. We have pointed out that, by identifying health with satisfaction, resignation risks to be encouraged, that satisfaction would be confused with a state of "resignation." But we have also said that health must be constantly supported by society and the family, so that people with disabilities can express their full potential to the maximum to look at themselves with greater objectivity. With social and family help, patients are neither deluded for impossible future achievements, nor are they depressed for unattainable achievements. At the end, they get to know, endure, and value their own achievements. In short, there must be a constant social, economic, cultural, and medical support; if they miss, you cannot speak of freedom or of health. Based on social support, people can enhance their residual possibilities or—if they do not want to fight—surrender to dissatisfaction and pain: but at least they have had a chance.

12.2.1 Health vs. Loneliness in End-of-Life Processes

But isn't it too relativistic to speak of health as satisfaction? No, if we read correctly the second part of the definition, which explains that health must be supported, socially and emotionally (Fig. 12.1). Defining health as a "state of satisfaction, socially supported" can be useful to avoid considering health as a utopia and consequently feeling disappointed for the awareness of never being able to obtain it [10]. The person in a terminal state can do a certain series of things and will be paradoxically serene and satisfied if they can do at least those—for example, eating, drinking, having social relationships, remembering past things of course if this is their wish and do not desire anything else. Thus, despite always hard, the end of life can become something else than the antinomy of health. To get this goal, children must not remain alone in the grief of the disease, they must express as much as possible their full desires; the society and the family should allow this, allowing the personal potential of the minor with a disability to be expressed. The tragedy of some ethical positions is that they pretend to equate freedom and solitude though autonomy and self-determination are not free if they are lived in conditions of abandon or loneliness. Clark and Oates showed "a specific congruent interaction between Solitude, one of the two dimensions of autonomy, and negative autonomous events" [11]. Deciding alone on one's own health, leads to decisions not based on objective facts about one's own illness and one's potential, but on fear or illusion. It is rather to be done in a context of solidarity that leads to a balanced vision.

The concept of health, as we have outlined it, applies in a special way to the children. In fact, when can we say that a child with cancer lacks health?

In the case of children too young to realize that they are dying, grief and moral suffering are simply absent, their satisfaction will be intact, unless the reaction to grief and sadness or despair of their parents may surprise and make them suffer. Paradoxically, we can say that in these cases, lacking awareness defends from the conscience of illness and health is not undermined.

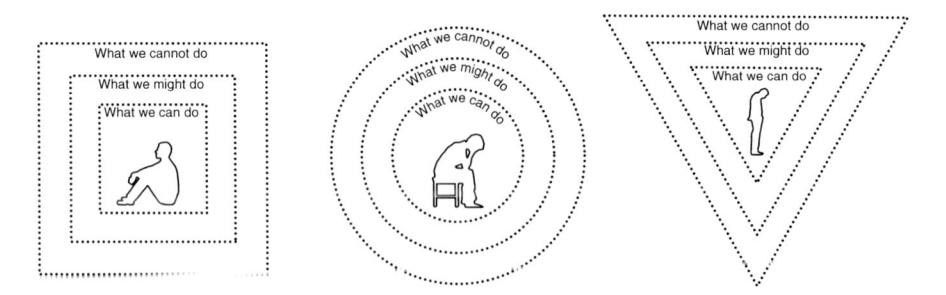

Fig. 12.1 Health is the personal satisfaction socially supported. Health is present when we are satisfied of what we can do, despite what we cannot and what we might do, and despite anyone has their own kind of things they can do (here represented by different geometric figures that surround each human body). But this satisfaction should be socially supported (see text). If there is no social support, there is loneliness, not health

In the case of an older child, who begins to understand and deal with the concept of death, things are different. The parental environment will be fundamental because death is still an abstract concept: the concept of death, the perspective of death is not a real perspective for them, so it will affect health only if the environment spills despair on the child, despair that does not come from inside of them.

For the adolescents, this is quite different: they have not yet a mature development of rationality, they are instinctive, sometimes they want to intimidate their friends. The idea of their well-being, of their satisfaction and therefore of their health is variable, without a long-term vision, without either a clear fear of death or much empathy with the parents with whom he is usually in conflict. So, their sense of health will depend upon the environment: their friends, influencers, and social networks. Nonetheless, these children have their desires, their wishes, and are deeply disappointed by knowing that wishes and desires will be only a dream: this undermines their satisfaction and health, until they get to accept this ineluctable event.

Pain, of course, changes everything. Physical pains disrupt any sense of satisfaction and health.

12.3 Supporting Mental Hygiene for a Really Free Choice

Performing free choices is fundamental in an end-of-life set, both in Intensive Pediatric Care Units and in Palliative Care Departments. Much of our free choices depends by the dynamic between our wishes and desires, and the superior instances of life, aka totems. Jacques Lacan was one of the most influential philosophers who correlated mental health with human desires [12]. Lacan focused his analysis of human mind on the concept of desire; for him, human desire is a metonymy [13], i.e., something that is not identified in a specific thing, that recalls or refers to something else. The human desire is a never-ending process of continual deferral; it is always "desire for something else" [14] as soon as the object of desire is attained, it is no longer desirable, and the subject's desire fixes on another object.

Echoing Sigmund Freud, we might argue that we all have our totems-desires in our life [15]. Totems are the supreme goals that we want to achieve. Totems can be survival, career, youth, absence of diseases, etc. To these totems, we give an important meaning in the achievement of happiness. To get these totems, each of us relies on intermediate desires or successes [16], to which the achievement of the totem is often inextricably linked; for example, passing a career exam to obtain the totem of social success, or having a certain physical appearance to achieve the totem of an always young life or a success in the sexual field. Or overcoming a sudden disease.

Thus, we have "desires" through which we suppose to arrive to the "totems," and totems through which we suppose to get happiness. When the object of the desires is not gotten, either because we cannot achieve them or because we have lost them, different feelings are triggered. But, as Lacan wrote, desire cannot be stuck in one object, our happiness cannot be signified by one object. Human neuroses, under the names of hysteric neurosis and obsessive neurosis, have in common the idealization

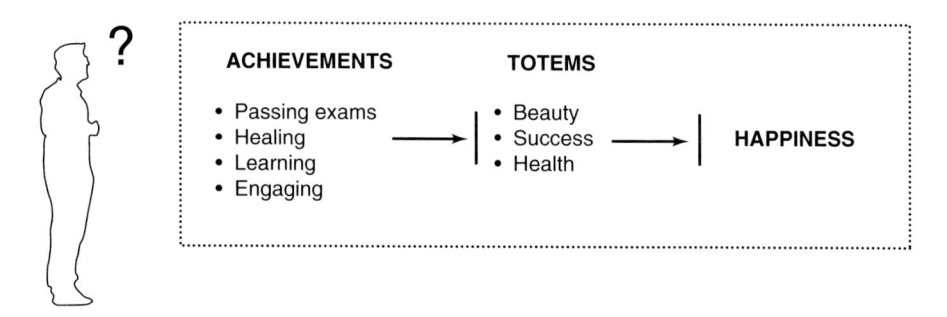

Fig. 12.2 The totems and achievements. There is usually a tight knot between achievements and totems, and totems and happiness. We should help unknot it

of the desire. Thus, a mental hygiene needs to obey to the law of the desire that shows it as a metonymy, i.e., not as a specific object and not as an absolute need.

This correlates with end-of-life and palliative care treatment, and will need to be managed by specialists. Because it is necessary to cut the link between "object of a desire" (the success of a test) and "totem" (such as the desire for health, for life, for beauty, for decreasing suffer); and to cut the link between "totem" and the achievement of happiness (Fig. 12.2). Otherwise, the patient will end in hurting themselves.

The first step (dissolving the link between achievement and the totem) helps the patient understand the distance and the equivocal correlation between a symptom or sign of illness and the loss of one totem such as health. Being sick does not necessarily mean that we cannot be healthy, as we have just seen. The second step is the most difficult since it consists of cutting the link between the totem (beauty, health) and happiness, that is, making it clear that you can be serene even when forces leave you, when beauty disappears, when your life ends. It is difficult, it is not always successful, but it is possible. We must help these children creating a roadmap with psychologists, physicians, and biologists. We must dissolve the equation between sickness and loss of health and between loss of health and unhappiness.

References

1. Conti AA. Historical evolution of the concept of health in Western medicine. Acta Biomed. 2018;89(3):352–4. https://doi.org/10.23750/abm.v89i3.6739.
2. Bellieni CV. Salute e Benessere, una definizione Nuova. Medicina e Morale. 2009;58(4).
3. Oleribe OO, Ukwedeh O, Burstow NJ, Gomaa AI, Sonderup MW, Cook N, Waked I, Spearman W, Taylor-Robinson SD. Health: redefined. Pan Afr Med J. 2018;30:292. https://doi.org/10.11604/pamj.2018.30.292.15436.
4. Jacobsen PL, Rudin RS. To your health. Keeping fit for life in dentistry. J Am Dent Assoc. 1991,122(12):49–52. https://doi.org/10.14219/jada.archive.1991.0188.
5. Svalastog AL, Donev D, Jahren Kristoffersen N, Gajović S. Concepts and definitions of health and health-related values in the knowledge landscapes of the digital society. Croat Med J. 2017;58(6):431–5. https://doi.org/10.3325/cmj.2017.58.431.

6. Pinto S, Fumincelli L, Mazzo A, Caldeira S, Martins JC. Comfort, well-being and quality of life: discussion of the differences and similarities among the concepts. Porto Biomed J. 2017;2(1):6–12. https://doi.org/10.1016/j.pbj.2016.11.003. Epub 2017 Jan 1.
7. Lulé D, Zickler C, Häcker S, Bruno MA, Demertzi A, Pellas F, Laureys S, Kübler A. Life can be worth living in locked-in syndrome. Prog Brain Res. 2009;177:339–51. https://doi.org/10.1016/S0079-6123(09)17723-3.
8. Zheng QL, Tian Q, Hao C, Gu J, Lucas-Carrasco R, Tao JT, Liang ZY, Chen XL, Fang JQ, Ruan JH, Ai QX, Hao YT. The role of quality of care and attitude towards disability in the relationship between severity of disability and quality of life: findings from a cross-sectional survey among people with physical disability in China. Health Qual Life Outcomes. 2014;12:25. https://doi.org/10.1186/1477-7525-12-25.
9. Krahn GL, Robinson A, Murray AJ, Havercamp SM. Nisonger RRTC on Health and Function. It's time to reconsider how we define health: perspective from disability and chronic condition. Disabil Health J. 2021;14(4):101129.
10. Sartorius N. The meanings of health and its promotion. Croat Med J. 2006;47(4):662–4.
11. Clark DA, Oates T. Daily hassles, major and minor life events, and their interaction with sociotropy and autonomy. Behav Res Ther. 1995;33(7):819–23. https://doi.org/10.1016/0005-7967(95)00020-x.
12. De Battista J. Lacanian Concept of Desire in Analytic Clinic of Psychosis. Front Psychol. 2017;8:563. https://doi.org/10.3389/fpsyg.2017.00563.
13. Lacan J. Écrits: a selection. Trans. Alan Sheridan. London: Tavistock Publications; 1977b. p. 167.
14. Lacan J. Écrits: a selection, transl. by Alan Sheridan. New York: W.W. Norton & Co.; 1977a.
15. Grossman WI. Freud's presentation of 'the psychoanalytic mode of thought' in Totem and taboo and his technical papers. Int J Psychoanal. 1998;79(Pt 3):469–86.
16. Pettit P. Desire—Routledge encyclopedia of philosophy. www.rep.routledge.com. Accessed 4 May 2021.

Children and Babies: Decisions on Their Health

13.1 Treating Every Newborn at All Costs?

We premise that an extremely vitalistic approach to this problem should be avoided. Doctors and parents should be aware that limits to the possibilities of the modern medicine exist, and that children do not have to undergo useless, futile, or painful treatments without consistent hopes of improvement. A recent review [1] has summarized the guidelines to be followed in neonatal resuscitation, in vogue in several countries. The authors show that most Western countries are far from the risk of vitalism; on the contrary, resuscitation is subordinated to gestational age, if babies are born below a certain threshold that does not coincide with that of viability, but with that of likelihood (not certainty) of brain damage. Moreover, this review shows that in these preterm babies, much of the decision relies on the parents, who can allow or prohibit resuscitation. This happens with the aim of avoiding unnecessary suffering and a future disability; nonetheless, a Swedish study by Stellån Hakansson and others [2] showed that neonatal resuscitation units where a selection at birth is performed on the basis of the likelihood of becoming disabled, paradoxically end up having more disabled children than other units. This is counterintuitive, since it seems likely that whoever selects the most adapted to live will have fewer future disabilities but this study shows that the opposite is true. This could be due to the fact that, by making this selection at birth, one undergoes the risk of placing the "interest of third parties" (see [3]) as a criterion for resuscitation; or to the fact that even those who will not be really disabled are overselected and deprived of cures.

Birth at less than 25 weeks of gestation is often considered a "gray area," in which active treatments must occur exceptionally (according to some) only with the agreement of the parents, despite the fact that the survival rate of these children increases year after year [4]. Resuscitating children who have a 10% chance of survival is said to be excessive. We should reflect on this: in the 1970s, when a child weighing less than a pound had a 10% chance of survival, no one thought that intervening actively on these babies was therapeutical excess, and this has led to the

© The Author(s), under exclusive license to Springer Nature Switzerland AG 2022
C. V. Bellieni, *A New Holistic-Evolutive Approach to Pediatric Palliative Care*, https://doi.org/10.1007/978-3-030-96256-2_13

survival of many newborns, though several of these with disability, and to improve neonatal care, so that now the chances of survival when born with less than one pound of weight are 90%. There is much to discuss and progress together with all neonatologists in this field.

The non-resuscitation of the small patients also creates problems on a scientific level.

First, at birth there is no certainty about the prognosis; therefore, when it is proposed not to actively treat children born before a certain gestational age, this happens in a probabilistic, statistical way (also notice that the exact age from conception is usually at least questionable).

Second, about 15% of children born 22 weeks after conception could survive, a percentage equal to that of adults who survive cardiac arrest, whom no one, at the moment, proposes not to rescue, even though after a cardiac arrest they risk severe brain damage. Notice that the neurological consequences in these small preterm babies are not always devastating although in many cases there are serious disabilities as a consequence of premature birth. In 2005, Marlow reported that 22% of survivors under 25 weeks will have a severe disability, 24% a medium disability and 34% a mild disability at the age of 6 years of age [5]. A German study by Jochen Steinmacher [6] shows that 57% of survivors among those born 23–25 weeks after conception go to school regularly. They are better data than the prognosis of an adult suffering a stroke that the doctor has the obligation, and not the option, to treat.

Third, many authors propose that parents play a decisive role in making decisions about their children's life. But deliveries are often rushed (the woman is obviously in the midst of painful contractions and the father could be highly stressed, so neither of them would have the serenity to think) and it is not possible to take decisions with an information obtained in few instants, on things that require years of study to be competent on them; moreover, parents may have a conflict of interests when deciding between their baby's survival or the chance of taking care of a disabled child for years.

Some authors question why the way of treating newborns is different from other patients. In fact, no adult would be withdrawn from treatment if the prognosis was not certain, and no one would think of not trying to cure them if the chances of success were low; however, this happens with premature babies [3, 7].

The analysis of scientific studies shows something else. In fact, it is clear that behind an apparent rational criterion of withdrawing treatments in the "best interests of the patient," it may lie the fears and anxieties of the physicians themselves, rather than a clinically objective criterion. A 2007 Australian study showed that neonatologists who resuscitate the least are the most fearful of getting sick and dying [8]. Other studies show that the age, sex, religion, ethnicity of the doctor, and the presence of disabled people in the family have an influence on the life and death decisions that the patient will make. A study by Annie Janvier [9] shows the level of this prejudice: when asking a group of doctors if they would resuscitate a baby born at 24 weeks of gestational age, only 21% answered affirmatively; when asked if they would resuscitate an adult patient with a 50% risk of death and a 25% risk of disability, the percentage rises to 51%. But this forecast is exactly equivalent to the forecast for babies born at 24 weeks. That is, they would resuscitate an adult with this prognosis but not a baby with the same prognosis.

13.2 Shifting Too Soon to Palliative Care

A subordinate risk is the shift of these babies to palliative treatments with the withdrawal of intensive care, when they are not terminal, but when a future poor quality of life is likely [10]. This would never happen in the case of an older child or of an adult. So, we should watch over that the emotively good proposal of palliative care, that is always better than no treatment, does not overshadow a too quick and only partially motivated suspension of vital efforts.

13.3 Prejudices Against Disabled Children

Disability has always been subject to discrimination [11]. Speaking of palliative care, disabled people have a clear risk: that the decision to suspend care in the case of acute or chronic illness, will concern them with greater liberality than people without apparent disabilities. The possibility of a hidden euthanasia has been described [12]. This may be due to philosophical reasons:

- Subjects with disabilities are not considered by some scholars to be full persons, so the care they receive is not equal to that of the rest of the population. Some think that in order to be defined as "people" one must show clear self-determination, that many disabled people do not possess, as we will see elsewhere in this book [13].
- We can consider that the disabled people are a burden to the family and see them only and exclusively in this light; therefore, allowing them to die without giving them all the possibilities that an average person may receive would be an act of little gravity since it would take away a burden from a family that is often economically and psychologically burdened by the presence of the patient.
- It can be considered that the presence of the disabled person is a high social cost that is not justified by the benefits that the disabled person brings to society or that he brings to himself as a subject of low intellectual capacity and apparently not able to enjoy the benefits of life. Various proposals were recently done by some governments to limit access to intensive care in the event of COVID to those who have a better chance of having a benefit from continuing life, excluding from intensive care the elderly [14] and severely disabled people [15].

The prejudices shown about the disabled are evident. There are prejudices towards the condition of the disabled, and the first is that he cannot enjoy life, that the quality of life is necessarily low and that it is a burden to the family in a serious and disastrous way. Nonetheless, the quality of life of the disabled person is not necessarily low [16]; the family of the disabled person would like to have more aid from the State, rather than to think of having their family member die [17]; the disabled person has his own personal way of enjoying the things and experiences that life offers them, obviously in a special way.

Of course, we shouldn't even indulge to pietism. We cannot believe every life to be bearable both by the sick person and by the family.

References

1. Pignotti MS, Berni R. Extremely preterm births: end-of-life decisions in European countries. Arch Dis Child Fetal Neonatal Ed. 2010;95(4):F273–6. https://doi.org/10.1136/adc.2009.168294. Epub 2010 Apr 13.
2. Håkansson S, Farooqi A, Holmgren PA, Serenius F, Högberg U. Proactive management promotes outcome in extremely preterm infants: a population-based comparison of two perinatal management strategies. Pediatrics. 2004;114(1):58–64. https://doi.org/10.1542/peds.114.1.58.
3. Gross ML. Abortion and neonaticide: ethics, practice, and policy in four nations. Bioethics. 2002;16(3):202–30. https://doi.org/10.1111/1467-8519.00282.
4. Fanaroff JM, Hascoët JM, Hansen TW, Levene M, Norman M, Papageorgiou A, Shinwell E, van de Bor M, Stevenson DK. International Perinatal Collegium (IPC). The ethics and practice of neonatal resuscitation at the limits of viability: an international perspective. Acta Paediatr. 2014;103(7):701–8. https://doi.org/10.1111/apa.12633. Epub 2014 Apr 3.
5. Marlow N, Wolke D, Bracewell MA, Samara M, EPICure Study Group. Neurologic and developmental disability at six years of age after extremely preterm birth. N Engl J Med. 2005;352(1):9–19. https://doi.org/10.1056/NEJMoa041367.
6. Steinmacher J, Pohlandt F, Bode H, Sander S, Kron M, Franz AR. Neurodevelopmental follow-up of very preterm infants after proactive treatment at a gestational age of > or = 23 weeks. J Pediatr. 2008;152(6):771–6, 776.e1–2. https://doi.org/10.1016/j.jpeds.2007.11.004. Epub 2008 Jan 22.
7. Janvier A, Barrington KJ, Payot A. A time for hope: guidelines for the perinatal management of extremely preterm birth. Arch Dis Child Fetal Neonatal Ed. 2020;105(3):230–1. https://doi.org/10.1136/archdischild-2019-318553. Epub 2020 Mar 10.
8. Barr P. Relationship of neonatologists' end-of-life decisions to their personal fear of death. Arch Dis Child Fetal Neonatal Ed. 2007;92(2):F104–7. https://doi.org/10.1136/adc.2006.094151. Epub 2007 Feb 6.
9. Janvier A, Lantos J, Deschênes M, Couture E, Nadeau S, Barrington KJ. Caregivers attitudes for very premature infants: what if they knew? Acta Paediatr. 2008;97(3):276–9. https://doi.org/10.1111/j.1651-2227.2008.00663.x.
10. Janvier A, Farlow B, Verhagen E, Barrington K. End-of-life decisions for fragile neonates: navigating between opinion and evidence-based medicine. Arch Dis Child Fetal Neonatal Ed. 2017;102(2):F96–F97.
11. Schmidt-Michel PO, Müller T. Der Umgang mit Angehörigen der Opfer der Aktion "T4" durch die NS-Behörden und die Anstalten in Württemberg [Dealing with Relatives of the Victims of the "Aktion T4" by the National Socialist Institutions as well as by Wuerttemberg Asylums]. Psychiatr Prax. 2018;45(3):126–32. https://doi.org/10.1055/s-0044-100193. Epub 2018 Jan 23.
12. Spreeuwenberg C. Dutch higher court places further limitations on physician-assisted death. Int J Integr Care. 2002;2:e06. https://doi.org/10.5334/ijic.47.
13. United Nations, International Covenant on Civil and Political Rights Concluding observations of the Human Rights Committee: Netherlands. Paras 5–6. (CCPR/CO/72/NET.); 2001. http://www.unhchr.ch/tbs/doc.nsf/(Symbol)/CCPR.CO.72.NET.En?Opendocument. Accessed 21 Mar 2005.

14. Cardoso FS, Borges A, Botelho I, Real A, Araújo AC, Domingos G, Pereira R, Moreno R, Bento L, Germano N. Access to Intensive Care Unit Care for elderly patients with COVID-19 in Portugal. Port J Public Health. 2020;38:91–3. https://doi.org/10.1159/000511150.
15. Riva L, Petrini C. Ethics of triage for intensive-care interventions during the COVID-19 pandemic: age or disability related cut-off policies are not justifiable. Clin Ethics. 2020. https://doi.org/10.1177/1477750920971803.
16. Mayer RCF, Alves MR, Yamauti SM, Silva MT, Lopes LC. Quality of life and functioning of people with mental disorders who underwent deinstitutionalization using assisted living facilities: a cross-sectional study. Front Psychol. 2021;12:622973. https://doi.org/10.3389/fpsyg.2021.622973.
17. Wright Stein S, Alexander R, Mann J, Schneider C, Zhang S, Gibson BE, Gabison S, Jachyra P, Mosleh D. Understanding disability in healthcare: exploring the perceptions of parents of young people with autism spectrum disorder. Disabil Rehabil. 2021;1–8.

The Pain Principle

14.1 Therapeutic Fury

An important dilemma in children's care is avoiding excesses in treatment. Sometimes, invasively painful or useless treatments should be removed. To this aim, we should be aware of what "useless" really means, and reflect that sometimes "futile treatments" are erroneously identified with those displayed to save a life with poor features. This is an abuse, though we should be aware that excessively "vitalistic" principles should be rejected, namely those that want to save lives at all costs, even against the interest of the patient of avoiding suffering.

In some countries, the concept of "therapeutic fury" has been introduced. It is commonly confused with that of "futile treatments". Here we use the term "therapeutic fury" used in Latin-derived languages, where it reminds the harassment of an animal on a pree ("accanimento" in Italian, "encharnement" in French, "ensanamiento" in Spanish). The concept of therapeutic fury does not deal with those treatments manifestly ineffective, but those that provoke further suffering, just as an aggressive animal might do. Defining what "therapeutic fury" is, has always been a big problem. For some, the therapeutic cruelty may be when we allow the survival of a severely disabled child, but this runs up against the right of any citizen to treatment, regardless of their pathology, race, religion, or behavior; therefore, we need a serious and verifiable criterion. But therapeutic fury is not simply the use of ineffective treatments (common sense is enough for avoiding that); we can define it as "any treatment that, without giving any benefit, determines or exacerbates stress and/or pain documented in the subject, and without a free acceptance of this pain" [1]. If it does not provoke pain, it is not excessive, but it is simply futile. This definition has three corollaries:

1. Assessing pain. Ineffective treatments that do not generate pain and stress, are not "fierceness" (which presupposes harm to the subject), but simply do not make sense.
2. No benefit. The stress/pain caused to the child can in some cases be unavoidable but useful to cure them, so we would not speak of therapeutic fierceness. In this case, however, a criterion of proportionality [2] should be used in relation to two factors: the level of pain/stress inflicted and the utility for the subject. For example, in the child with extreme irreversible brain damage (affecting the relationship life), the level of pain/stress that our treatments can cause must be minimal since the treatments themselves (resuscitation attempts, surgery, etc.) will hardly benefit the child, due to his pathology that does not allow him to enjoy real life [3].
3. Not accepted. Adults may ask to continue certain treatments because they feel they can bear the pain, to ward off and procrastinate death according to their will. That is not the case with a baby; the baby cannot choose to endure the pain, so the pain is presumed not accepted and while an adult can accept a painful and useless treatment, the baby cannot, and should not be given, unless the benefit it gives is utterly evident and beneficial.

In the case of intense and intractable stress/pain, the invasiveness of the treatments can be reduced by implementing palliative care.

We will here propose an easy way to help physicians take the best decision in end-of-life matters. It is the "Pain Principle." It is not an absolute criterion but is utterly useful. Before describing the pain principle, we will review the main principle that are applied currently, before introducing and describing the pain principle.

14.2 The Best Interest Principle and Its Limitations

One criterion that is often proposed for suspending or continuing intensive pediatric care is the so-called best interest principle [4]: trying to act in the best interest of the patient. The problem is: who really knows the best interest of a non-verbal baby or child? What is sure is that sometimes even adults are not sure about what constitutes their own best interest. We have recently seen cases in which both those who wanted to suspend a treatment and those who wanted to continue it appealed to the criterion of best interest, thus showing the intrinsic weakness of this principle that can be used at the same time in favor or against a treatment [5].

The best interest of the child represents the guiding principle of all the legislation for the protection of the child, ensuring that in all decisions concerning the child, the judge must take into account the best interests of the child. For example, the principle of best interest finds great application in the case of the custody of the minor to a parent after a separation or divorce. However, there remains a series of doubts about this principle.

14.3 The Probabilistic Criterion

One criterion followed to resuscitate newborns is the probabilistic criterion: in the first few days or hours of life, it has not yet been possible to make a sure diagnosis and prognosis of brain damage; therefore, several protocols suggest a selective resuscitation depending on the pregnancy time when the baby was born, since the birth at a certain gestational age corresponds to a particular prognosis. This criterion has been the object of various criticisms [6]. As we have seen, Annie Janvier's studies on the decisions at the end of life in neonatology lead to worrying conclusions: babies in several countries are being resuscitated or not resuscitated with different decision criteria than those with which similar decisions are made about older children. Other studies show how, within the same country, newborns are resuscitated with more or less interventionist criteria depending on the area and that in the same hospital, newborns, and pediatric patients receive substantially different resuscitations to the detriment of the former.

14.4 The Double Effect

A criterion to always keep in mind is that of the "double effect." Its basis is the following: if the aim is to cure or relieve pain, and in the attempt to achieve this goal there is a risk of shortening the patient's life, this risk is ethically legitimate, because none wants to voluntarily cause death; and if this occurs, this happens as a part of an attempt made in the patient's interest [7, 8].

This doctrine considers the mixture of good and evil as a consequence of human action. It must be established to what extent, respecting our duties, we can cause evil along with good.

The "double effect" principle features two main points to make an action acceptable:

1. The act must be morally good or at least indifferent.
2. The good purpose must be evident, while the bad one must only be foreseen or tolerated, but not directly intended.

14.5 The Least Harm Criterion

The best interest criterion was criticized in particular by Douglas Diekema of the University of Washington, who preferred to replace it with the so-called harm principle: it is much easier to know (and eliminate) what causes the harm, than to know the interest of the patient [9]. The harm principle provides a foundation for interfering with parental choices when they seem unreasonable, and more in detail, it describes an appropriate standard for interfering with parents who refuse to consent to medical treatment on behalf of a child. According to the harm principle, State intervention is justified not when a parental refusal is contrary to a child's best interest, but when the parental refusal places the child at significant risk of serious preventable harm.

14.6 The Pain Principle

Nonetheless, the concept of harm is also vague and, often, indeterminate (there is moral, physical, economic harm, etc.). Therefore, based on Diekema's observations, another approach can be considered in end-of-life decisions: the "pain principle," according to which, whether treatments cause uncontrollable pain, then and only then can they be gradually reduced in intensity: it is unethical to continue causing severe pain [3] to those who cannot freely accept it because they are very small, fragile and mute, if they will not have a benefit from it. The advantage of this principle is that pain, unlike "interest" or "harm," can be measured with laboratory tools available to the clinicians.

In 2016, several scientific Societies issued a statement according to which "ICU interventions should generally be considered inappropriate when there is no reasonable expectation that the patient will improve sufficiently to survive outside the acute care setting, or when there is no reasonable expectation that the patient's neurologic function will improve sufficiently to allow the patient to perceive the benefits of treatment" [10]. Some questions can be raised about the first part of this definition: a patient in ICU is still a patient and a person; this is not deleted just by their being in ICU. The second part is interesting because it invites to consider the level of perception of the patient: a severely brain-damaged patient will not get any advantage from a painful procedure.

Nowadays, the pain and stress that a child suffers and cannot express, can be measured in several ways: with electronic instruments [11], with the evaluation of the production of stress hormones (e.g. cortisol levels either in blood or saliva) [12], and with multifactorial scales [13, 14]. To assess pain, the variability of the heart rate or the conductance of the skin can be measured, both signals of activation of the autonomic nervous system [15, 16]. It is even possible to perform electroencephalographic brain mapping to see the presence of activation of the areas that are switched on in case of stress and pain [17].

Objectivity is important, to evaluate the data and not the impressions; we should not judge that "maybe" the baby is feeling pain, since we have tools to know the state of stress. It would be atrocious to suspend a treatment thinking that the patients are suffering, when in reality they are not, just as it would be atrocious to let someone suffer because we are not realizing that suffering is present. With intractable stress or pain, the treatments that cause them must be changed or reduced, not in order to kill, but to reduce the suffering they cause.

The pain principle (Fig. 14.1) helps clinicians to avoid excessive vitalism, that wants to save lives at all costs, and a too early shift from proactive to palliative care.

This criterion has a two-point corollary.

(a) When babies have no benefit from the cures, namely when their mental damage will not allow any level of social interaction, no pain should be allowed and treatments that provoke it should be withdrawn.
(b) When a mental level of social interaction still exists, a proportional level of pain—when unavoidable and useful to the baby's improvement—can be allowed.

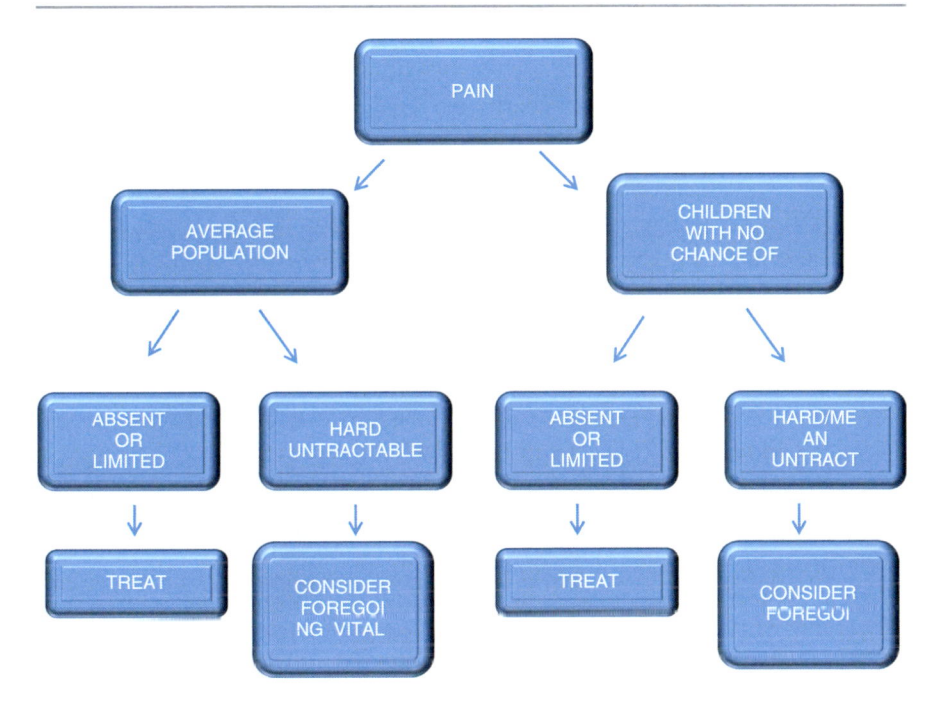

Fig. 14.1 The pain principle

Notice that when we predict with certainty a future unavoidable pain, the points (a) and (b) can be taken into consideration: the pain principle does not concern only present pain, but also future, if sure and ineluctable, pain.

References

1. Bellieni CV, Buonocore G. Using the pain principle to provide a new approach to invasive treatments and end-of-life care. Acta Paediatr. 2019;108(2):206–7. https://doi.org/10.1111/apa.14535. Epub 2018 Sep 17.
2. Picozzi M, Pegoraro R. Taking care of the vulnerable: the criterion of proportionality. Am J Bioeth. 2017;17(8):44–5. https://doi.org/10.1080/15265161.2017.1340997.
3. Bellieni C. The pain principle: an ethical approach to end-of-life decisions. Ethics Med. 2020;36(1):41–9.
4. Spence K. The best interest principle as a standard for decision making in the care of neonates. J Adv Nurs. 2000;31(6):1286–92. https://doi.org/10.1046/j.1365-2648.2000.01402.x.
5. Jonas M, Ryan S. The discourse of dignity in the Charlie Gard, Alfie Evans and Isaiah Haastrup Cases. Med Law Rev. 2020;29(1):24–47. https://doi.org/10.1093/medlaw/fwaa038. Epub ahead of print.
6. Janvier A, Farlow B, Verhagen E, Barrington K. End-of-life decisions for fragile neonates: navigating between opinion and evidence-based medicine. Arch Dis Child Fetal Neonatal Ed. 2017;102(2):F96–F97.
7. Potter J, Shields S, Breen R. Palliative sedation, compassionate extubation, and the principle of double effect: an ethical analysis. Am J Hosp Palliat Care. 2021;38(12):1536–40. https://doi.org/10.1177/1049909121998630. Epub ahead of print.
8. Reed PA. Opioids, double effect, and the prospects of hastening death. J Med Philos. 2021;46(5):505–15. https://doi.org/10.1093/jmp/jhab016. Epub ahead of print.

9. Diekema DS. Parental refusals of medical treatment: the harm principle as threshold for state intervention. Theor Med Bioeth. 2004;25(4):243–64. https://doi.org/10.1007/s11017-004-3146-6.
10. Kon AA, Shepard EK, Sederstrom NO, Swoboda SM, Marshall MF, Birriel B, Rincon F. Defining futile and potentially inappropriate interventions: a policy statement from the Society of Critical Care Medicine Ethics Committee. Crit Care Med. 2016;44(9):1769–74. https://doi.org/10.1097/CCM.0000000000001965.
11. Benoit B, Martin-Misener R, Newman A, Latimer M, Campbell-Yeo M. Neurophysiological assessment of acute pain in infants: a scoping review of research methods. Acta Paediatr. 2017;106(7):1053–66. https://doi.org/10.1111/apa.13839. Epub 2017 May 9.
12. Shetty V, Suresh LR, Hegde AM. Effect of virtual reality distraction on pain and anxiety during dental treatment in 5 to 8 year old children. J Clin Pediatr Dent. 2019;43(2):97–102. https://doi.org/10.17796/1053-4625-43.2.5. Epub 2019 Feb 7.
13. Beltramini A, Milojevic K, Pateron D. Pain assessment in newborns, infants, and children. Pediatr Ann. 2017;46(10):e387–95. https://doi.org/10.3928/19382359-20170921-03.
14. Jain AA, Yeluri R, Munshi AK. Measurement and assessment of pain in children—a review. J Clin Pediatr Dent. 2012;37(2):125–36. https://doi.org/10.17796/jcpd.37.2.k84341490806t770.
15. Chiera M, Cerritelli F, Casini A, Barsotti N, Boschiero D, Cavigioli F, Corti CG, Manzotti A. Heart rate variability in the perinatal period: a critical and conceptual review. Front Neurosci. 2020;14:561186. https://doi.org/10.3389/fnins.2020.561186.
16. Strehle EM, Gray WK. Comparison of skin conductance measurements and subjective pain scores in children with minor injuries. Acta Paediatr. 2013;102(11):e502–6. https://doi.org/10.1111/apa.12382. Epub 2013 Aug 30.
17. Garcia-Larrea L, Bastuji H. Pain and consciousness. Prog Neuro-Psychopharmacol Biol Psychiatry. 2018;87(Pt B):193–9. https://doi.org/10.1016/j.pnpbp.2017.10.007. Epub 2017 Oct 12.

Part V

The Multiple Approach to Suffering

This book has at its basis a synoptic view of the palliative care. This means that we should have an overall approach to children's pain. In fact, suffering is a complex phenomenon that includes psychological, physical, psychiatric and affective aspects, and the treatment of pain must be a global treatment as well, that includes them all. This also means that we want to be companions of the child in this difficult and hard passage of their lives, following and accompanying their steps. Here, we will describe the drugs used as analgesics and their adjuvants, but we also will deal with the prelude and precondition to all analgesic treatment, which consists of two points: a good environment and a good relationship with caregivers. So we are going to discuss of opioids and sedatives, of pain assessment, but also of psychological approaches to pain, of the importance of hospital setting and lodgments, and of doctors' stress and availability.

The Environment: The Base of Analgesic Efforts

15.1 Pain Is Not Just "Pain"

Pain produces in the patient hemodynamic alterations, changes of their internal metabolism and of respiratory patterns. It also produces fatigue, anxiety, insomnia, and feelings of loneliness. Pain generates disorders even in doctors and nurses: anxiety, frustration, fear, feeling of abandonment, fatigue. For these and many other reasons, pain management is an essential objective in pediatric palliative care. Pain is a fifth vital sign [1], and in some cases it can be considered a disease rather than a symptom [2]. Therefore, pain should be assessed, spotted, and cured, either chemically or psychologically.

Several drugs and analgesic treatments exist to overcome all this. Nonetheless, the first tool to cure pain is the environment: the surrounding conditions can enhance pain and suffering, while a positive environment can reduce pain sensation. We should detect and cure pain, but this cure cannot be just providing the right analgesic at the right moment and at the correct doses. Holding the child in a depressing and creepy room, without parents, pets, with rigid times for feeding or tidying up is the prelude to impairment. Usually, it is believed that the best healthcare is that which optimizes times and spaces and that gets the optimal cost/benefits rate, in a sort of "essential medicine" whose aim is making diagnoses and giving drugs [3]. This is wrong. A medicine of abundance is what is needed [4]. "Medicine of abundance" is the approach that puts at its center the improvement of the lifestyle and of the environment, both for the patients and of the personnel; it is a solid basis for drug treatment: without a solid basis, all treatments slip away on fragile sands. For instance, there is evidence to support the use of music in healing settings, in order to reduce pain and anxiety and improve the quality of life of children undergoing cancer treatment [5]; there is evidence that encourages pet therapy [6] or the well-known interventions of humor and laughter with hospital clowns [7]. All these

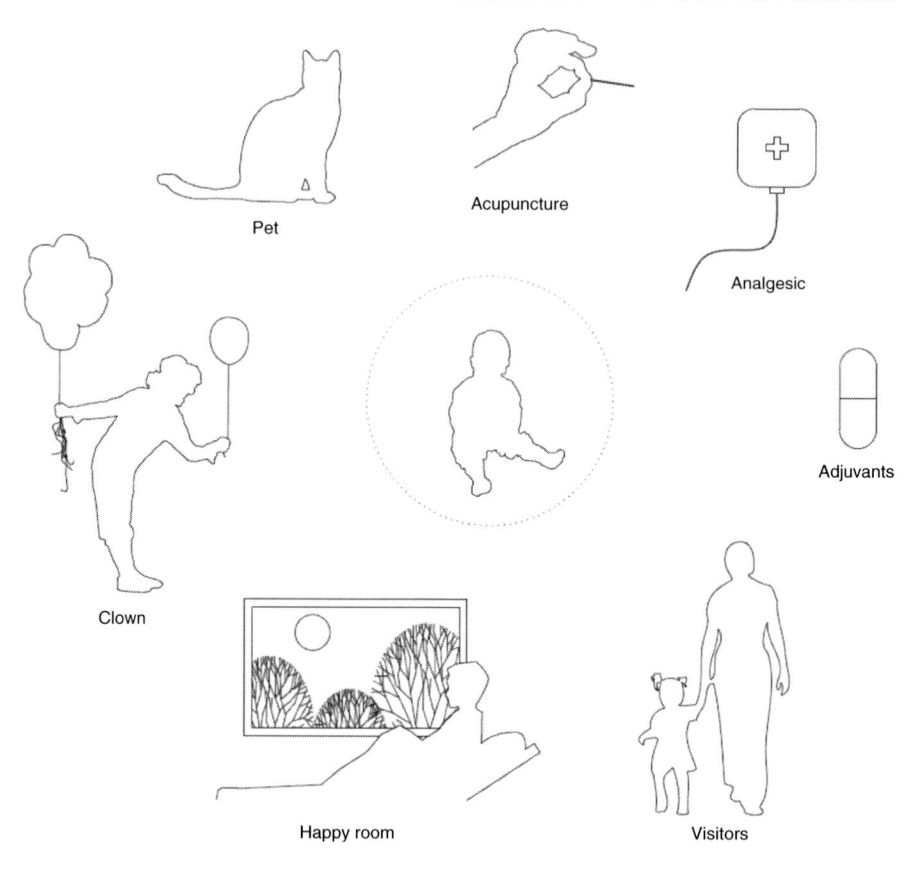

Fig. 15.1 The approach to children's pain is not limited only to the use of painkillers, but it deals with several other aspects of their life, starting from a serene environment, up to alternative medicines, non-pharmacological analgesia, and psychological-behavioral interventions

treatments are the stable basis for drug treatment; they enhance and increase the effect of analgesics (Fig. 15.1). Therefore, pain is not only pain, and analgesia is not only the administration of painkillers. Abundance is what is needed.

15.2 The Hospital as an Analgesic Tool

A joyful environment is somehow analgesic. It puts the basis of a good relationship between doctors and children, of better compliance and of more prompt recovery from illness. Therefore, the hospital is not neutral to the healing process and to the pain experience. A sad hospital increases the experience of sorrow, a vivid hospital improves the mood. So, several points should be guaranteed to make the hospital pain-free. Here, we express some of them; in the next paragraphs, others will be described in detail.

Continuity in activities: The child must be always considered as a child, they must continue their growth path, even during hospitalization; for this, they are involved in meaningful experiences, which strengthen their self-esteem and help them defeat their fears, soliciting positive energies useful for healing: illness and hospitalization should not only be a sad experience.

Presence of parents and friends: The modern "open wards" are organized with less strict rules than a few years ago, with regard to the visits of external people, so that every child and infant can enjoy the presence, next to them, of their parents, or at least of the mother: such contact is an indisputable need both for the child, who feels protected and reassured by family figures, and for the parents themselves, who at least would experience the disease in a participatory way. However, this important milestone may have to overcome the resistance of the prejudices sometimes opposed to the presence in the ward of adults familiar to the child, longtime considered intrusive and disturbing. Furthermore, from the 1960s onward, advances in hospital architecture have radically changed family housing to semi-private and private rooms [8] making it impossible for hospital staff to keep an eye on everything that happens next to the child, but guaranteeing their privacy.

Harmony: The child and their family must perceive the harmony among health workers: the sense of mistrust caused by the discrepancy among workers can lead to a decrease in compliance and to increase suffering and anxiety. In this search for harmony, pediatric hospices represent an important focal point: if the staff is truly motivated as they should, they act as an ideal bridge between the hospital and the home [9].

Continuity with domestic life: Urie Brofenbrenner's "Theory of ecological systems" [10] can be effectively applied to the relationships that are intertwined during the hospital experience and can become an interesting explanatory model. According to Brofenbrenner's theory, the child's development environment is a series of concentric circles, connected to each other by relationships. The child and his parents belong to two main microsystems: one refers to the personal context in which they are immersed in daily life and which directly influences them (common realities, work, relationships with friends, relatives, communities) and a second is that of the hospital context, in which they have to live and where they come in contact with other people (other parents, volunteers, medical and nursing staff, psychologists, educators, teachers). The set of relationships between microsystems (called mesosystem) is extremely important because it connects the world of the family with the world of the hospital. This theory on the house-hospital-child-family-staff interdependence is the substance of the patient's interpersonal relationships. One environment must not exclude the other. In particular, for the child with cancer it is essential that their family is able to maintain a good connection between the two microsystems: the family world (home) and the world of the disease (hospital); all subjects—the child, doctors, and parents—have the task of creating a bridge that connects these two worlds, a "vital and essential mesosystem for a good quality of life for the patient" [11].

15.2.1 Pet-Assisted Therapy

Animal-assisted therapy is a complementary strategy with an increasing presence in the literature. Limited studies have been conducted with children, particularly those with life-threatening and life-limiting conditions. Although outcomes are promising in decreasing suffering of children receiving palliative care services, more work is needed to validate evidence for the implementation of animal-assisted therapy with this vulnerable population [12]. Pet therapy is not so negligible as it is usually thought: several children have their favorite pet, and they can find great advantage in the presence of a non-pretentious and non-judging friendly companion. Mary Kaminsky and coll performed a study measuring saliva cortisol in a cohort of hospitalized children who received either pet therapy or another type of consolation (playing games, cards, videogames); the result was that the group of pet therapy disclosed less stress than the other one [13]. Having a dog in common life, decreases the anxiety due to social stressors in preadolescents [14]. Patients in Palliative Care Department have received important help by the presence of pet therapy: an Italian study reported how pets are safe and useful for hospitalized children, under the condition of an adequate training of the staff [15]. Clinical trials reported the usefulness of pet therapy against pain [16, 17]. A recent review reported that pet therapy improves mood and pain perception [18].

15.2.2 Clown Therapy

Laughter and humor fulfill one of the main goals of hospice palliative care: improving patients' overall quality of life [19]. Humor is an important aspect in pediatric palliative care. Shared laughter is a communication enhancer. Humor and laughter are useful in establishing the relationship between caregivers, patients, and relatives. They help break the ice in tense situations, build confidence, and reduce fear [20]. Once the therapeutic relationship is established, they can become a powerful healing agent. Laughter has been psychologically considered "a safe and acceptable outlet for repressed emotions" [21]. It provides a positive reference point for caregivers and patients, strengthens self-esteem in both, and serves as a protective mechanism. Research psychologists Thorson and Powell [22] have developed a multidimensional scale of humor, which was distributed to a total of 326 men and women in the general population and matched it with a scale of anxiety about death. Their results indicated a negative correlation between death anxiety and use of humor. This finding suggests that humor is a positive mechanism for some individuals, which acts balancing anxiety in facing death. Herth [23], in a study carried out with terminally ill patients, had found similar findings.

Humor helps breed hope, creates a sense of perspective, and helps establish a person's understanding of him/herself and others. Terminal patients have multiple and changing symptoms and disabilities resulting from their underlying disease. Emotionally, they suffer losses and regrets, and fear uncertain results. Spiritually, they are struggling with the end of life. This is overwhelming, unless we found some strategies to preserve a social life, and humor is one of these. If humor has benefits as important as those suggested, we must consider its legitimacy in the care of the dying patient.

Clown therapy is a simple approach to the use of humor in hospitals. Children escorted by clowns reported lower levels of pain upon admittance, discharge, and 12-h post-surgery [24], while another study showed that clown therapy was able to reduce children's anxiety though not pain [25]. A third study evidenced that clown therapy decreased both anxiety and pain in children [26].

15.2.3 Noise-Free Hospital

It is not enough to provide the best technologies and therapies to promote well-being: especially for children with chronic diseases or with a terminal situation, the environment must be tailored on them, since neonatal to teen age [27]. Unfortunately, the hospital environment is full of environmental pollution due to an overload of lights and sounds [28] and flooded with operating hours that do not coincide with the child's rhythms. Even in the incubators newborns are exposed to intolerable noise levels [29]. Established sound and noise levels must not be exceeded in a hospital, as well as night lighting parameters. The WHO so stated: "For most spaces in hospitals, the critical effects are sleep disturbance, annoyance, and communication interference, including warning signals. The LAmax of sound events during the night should not exceed 40 dB(A) indoors. For ward rooms in hospitals, the guideline values indoors are 30dB LAeq, together with 40 dB LAmax during night. Since patients have less ability to cope with stress, the LAeq level should not exceed 35 dB in most rooms in which patients are being treated or observed. Attention should be given to the sound levels in intensive care units and operating theaters. Sound inside incubators may result in health problems for neonates, including sleep disturbance, and may also lead to hearing impairment" [30].

15.2.4 Meals and Child-Friendly Hospitals

Even the meals for children are rarely designed on their preferences, but they respond to corporate economic logic and, at best, to the criteria of a sufficient caloric supplementation. A modern hospital must find an answer to this. A child-friendly environment is a place where stress is prevented, and, reducing stressful stimuli, pain and suffering are reduced as well, prescribed therapies are better accepted; it is an important help in better and faster healing for those symptoms that can be overcome [31]. A serene environment increases the effectiveness of analgesic therapies and makes operations on the child easier. Several interventions have been proposed and implemented to make a hospital more suitable for children. The Council of Europe issued a charter for a child-friendly hospital (https://rm.coe.int/168046ccef). To this aim, some indispensable tools are: school in the hospital, pet therapy, clown therapy, spaces and gyms for relaxation and entertainment, movie-theaters or

Table 15.1 Guideline values for community noise in specific environments

Specific environment	Critical health effect(s)	Decibel
Dwlling, indoors…	Speech intelligibility and moderate annoyance, daytime and evening	35
Inside bedrooms	Sleep disturbance, night-time	30
Hospital, ward rooms, indoors	Sleep disturbance, night-time	30
	Sleep disturbance, daytime and evenings	30

Note: Noise levels can easily be assessed using dedicated noise meters, but also using smartphone apps easily available

television rooms or video games. Colored walls, in-room television, and background music if appropriate are desirable as well. We reiterate that the presence of parents is not an optional that the hospital offers, but a right of the minor: depriving them of their parents because there are no spaces equipped for them, is a subtle violence (Table 15.1).

References

1. Rogers MP, Kuo PC. Pain as the fifth vital sign. J Am Coll Surg. 2020;231(5):601–2. https://doi.org/10.1016/j.jamcollsurg.2020.07.508.
2. Raffaeli W, Arnaudo E. Pain as a disease: an overview. J Pain Res. 2017;10:2003–8. https://doi.org/10.2147/JPR.S138864.
3. Fritze J. Is healthcare budgeting ethically justifiable? Eur J Health Econ. 2001;2(1):26–30. http://www.jstor.org/stable/3570030. Accessed 11 July 11 2021.
4. Bellieni CV. Healthcare consumerism is a threat for health. Gazz Med Ital Arch per le Sci Med. 2019;178(7–8):560–2.
5. da Silva Santa IN, Schveitzer MC, Dos Santos MLBM, Ghelman R, Filho VO. MUSIC INTERVENTIONS IN PEDIATRIC ONCOLOGY: systematic review and meta-analysis. Complement Ther Med. 2021;59:102725.
6. Urbanski BL, Lazenby M. Distress among hospitalized pediatric cancer patients modified by pet-therapy intervention to improve quality of life. J Pediatr Oncol Nurs. 2012;29(5):272–82.
7. Sridharan K, Sivaramakrishnan G. Therapeutic clowns in pediatrics: a systematic review and meta-analysis of randomized controlled trials. Eur J Pediatr. 2016;175(10):1353–60. https://doi.org/10.1007/s00431-016-2764-0. Epub 2016 Sep 8. Erratum in: Eur J Pediatr. 2017;176(5):681–682.
8. Markel H. When hospitals kept children from parents. New York Times; 2008. https://www.nytimes.com/2008/01/01/health/01visi.html
9. Corr CA, Corr DM. Pediatric hospice care. Pediatrics. 1985;76(5):774–80.
10. Bronfenbrenner U. Ecological systems theory (1992). In: Bronfenbrenner U, editor. Making human beings human: bioecological perspectives on human development. Sage Publications; 2005. p. 106–73.
11. Tremolada M, Bonichini S, Pillon M, Schiavo S, Carli M. Eliciting adaptive emotions in conversations with parents of leukemic children receiving therapy. J Psychos Oncol. 2011;29:327–46. https://doi.org/10.1080/07347332.2011.563341.
12. Gilmer MJ, Baudino MN, Tielsch Goddard A, Vickers DC, Akard TF. Animal-assisted therapy in pediatric palliative care. Nurs Clin North Am. 2016;51(3):381–95. https://doi.org/10.1016/j.cnur.2016.05.007.
13. Kaminski M, Pellino T, Wish J. Play and pets: the physical and emotional impact of child-life and pet therapy on hospitalized children. Child Health Care. 2002;31(4):321–35.

References

14. Kerns KA, Stuart-Parrigon KL, Coifman KG, van Dulmen MHM, Koehn A. Pet dogs: does their presence influence preadolescents' emotional responses to a social stressor? Soc Dev. 2018;27(1):34–44. https://doi.org/10.1111/sode.12246. Epub 2017 May 15.
15. Caprilli S, Messeri A. Animal-assisted activity at A. Meyer Children's Hospital: a pilot study. Evid Based Complement Alternat Med. 2006;3(3):379–83. https://doi.org/10.1093/ecam/nel029. Epub 2006 Apr 2.
16. Barchas D, Melaragni M, Abraham H, Barchas E. The best medicine: personal pets and therapy animals in the hospital setting. Crit Care Nurs Clin North Am. 2020;32(2):167–90. https://doi.org/10.1016/j.cnc.2020.01.002. Epub 2020 Apr 8.
17. Fiori G, Marzi T, Bartoli F, Bruni C, Ciceroni C, Palomba M, Zolferino M, Corsi E, Galimberti M, Moggi Pignone A, Viggiano MP, Guiducci S, Calamai M, Matucci-Cerinic M. The challenge of pet therapy in systemic sclerosis: evidence for an impact on pain, anxiety, neuroticism and social interaction. Clin Exp Rheumatol. 2018;36(Suppl 113):135–41. Epub 2018 Sep 20.
18. Diniz Pinto K, Vieira de Souza CT, Benamor Teixeira ML, da Silveira F, Gouvêa MI. Animal assisted intervention for oncology and palliative care patients: a systematic review. Complement Ther Clin Pract. 2021;43:101347. https://doi.org/10.1016/j.ctcp.2021.101347. Epub 2021 Mar 4.
19. Claxton-Oldfield S, Bhatt A. Is There a Place for Humor in Hospice Palliative Care? Volunteers Say "Yes"! Am J Hosp Palliat Care. 2017;34(5):417–22. https://doi.org/10.1177/1049909116632214. Epub 2016 Feb 25.
20. Savage BM, Lujan HL, Thipparthi RR, DiCarlo SE. Humor, laughter, learning, and health! A brief review. Adv Physiol Educ. 2017;41(3):341–7. https://doi.org/10.1152/advan.00030.2017.
21. Astedt-Kurki P, Liukkonen A. Humour in nursing care. J Adv Nurs. 1994;20:183–8.
22. Thorson JA, Powell FC. Relationships of death anxiety and sense of humor. Psych Reports. 1993;72:1364–6.
23. Herth K. Contributions of humor as perceived by the terminally ill. J Assoc Pediatr Oncol Nurs. 1987;4:14–22.
24. Newman N, Kogan S, Stavsky M, Pintov S, Lior Y. The impact of medical clowns exposure over postoperative pain and anxiety in children and caregivers: an Israeli experience. Pediatr Rep. 2019;11(3):8165. https://doi.org/10.4081/pr.2019.8165.
25. Felluga M, Rabach I, Minute M, Montico M, Giorgi R, Lonciari I, Taddio A, Barbi E. A quasi randomized-controlled trial to evaluate the effectiveness of clowntherapy on children's anxiety and pain levels in emergency department. Eur J Pediatr. 2016;175(5):645–50. https://doi.org/10.1007/s00431-015-2688-0. Epub 2016 Jan 12.
26. Yun OB, Kim SJ, Jung D. Effects of a clown-nurse educational intervention on the reduction of postoperative anxiety and pain among preschool children and their accompanying parents in South Korea. J Pediatr Nurs. 2015;30(6):e89–99. https://doi.org/10.1016/j.pedn.2015.03.003. Epub 2015 Apr 13.
27. Sekyia SR. Organizational change: the implementation of children-friendly hospitals. Cien Saude Colet. 2010;15(Supl. 1):1263–73.
28. Carvalho WB, Pedreira ML, de Aguiar MA. Noise level in a pediatric intensive care unit. J Pediatr. 2005;81(6):495–8. https://doi.org/10.2223/JPED.1424.
29. Bellieni CV, Buonocore G, Pinto I, Stacchini N, Cordelli DM, Bagnoli F. Use of sound-absorbing panel to reduce noisy incubator reverberating effects. Biol Neonate. 2003;84(4):293–6. https://doi.org/10.1159/000073637.
30. Berglund B et al. for the Guidelines for community Noise. e WHO-expert task force meeting held in London, United Kingdom; 1999. https://www.who.int/docstore/peh/noise/Comnoise-1.pdf.
31. Yoder JC, Staisiunas PG, Meltzer DO, Knutson KL, Arora VM. Noise and sleep among adult medical inpatients: far from a quiet night. Arch Intern Med. 2012;172(1):68–70. https://doi.org/10.1001/archinternmed.2011.603.

Assessment of Pain, of Sedation, and of Refractory Symptoms

16.1 Pain Assessment

About 70% of palliative care unit patients present moderate-severe pain at some point [1], while more than 80% patients with an oncological disease will have severe pain [2]. Pain assessment in pediatric palliative care patients is complex for two reasons: the broad spectrum of pain etiology (see Table 16.1) and the great difficulty of recognizing pain in babies and children with mental disabilities.

Mentally disabled children, as well as the smallest babies, do not speak; they can manifest the pain due to the aforementioned causes, with a generic disorder or even with no signs. For this reason, it is easy for pain and the cause that provoked it, to remain undiagnosed. Nurses and doctors specifically trained to heal adults, when they work in pediatric palliative care can fail to diagnose a trivial disease, such as an otitis, or an appendicitis, but also they may unrecognize pain. Several reports have shown that this has ominous consequences: see on this issue the MENCAP report "death by indifference" (https://www.mencap.org.uk/sites/default/files/2016-06/DBIreport.pdf), presented at the British Parliament in 2016, where a series of cases of unrecognized and therefore lethal disease were described among mentally disabled children and adults.

The assessment of the intensity of pain can be performed with validated scales for pain. Analogical visual scales are useful in patients who can understand and communicate adequately (see Table 16.1). The caregiver who uses these scales invites the patient to point their finger on a line where different faces express happiness or pain; the patient should point their finger at the level of the pain they are experiencing. In non-verbal patients, scales are forcely multiparametric: since the baby cannot speak and since a single parameter in not specific enough, several parameters are scored together, to support the final score with the sum of single items. These items are clinical parameters such as heart rate, respiratory rate, facial expression, and level of consolability. Pain assessment performed with validated tools is a mandatory procedure: detecting pain is not so easy in infancy, and even

---

© The Author(s), under exclusive license to Springer Nature Switzerland AG 2022
C. V. Bellieni, *A New Holistic-Evolutive Approach to Pediatric Palliative Care*, https://doi.org/10.1007/978-3-030-96256-2_16

Table 16.1 Causes of pain in pediatric palliative care

Cancer patients [3]	Noncancer patients, mainly affected by neurological diseases [4]
Pleuritis and pleural effusion	Secondary to muscle contractures
Vascular compression	Spasticity
Distention of visceral capsules	Osteoarticular deformities
Muscle spasms	Displacement of the viscera due to severe scoliosis that produce severe gastroesophageal reflux, intestinal pseudo-obstruction, etc. associated or not with fracture
Lymphedema	Muscle spasms secondary to seizures
Intracranial hypertension	Central pain (e.g., secondary to thalamic involvement)
Root or spinal compression	Bedsores
Bone or nerve infiltration	Constipation
Punctures, placement, and canalization of catheters, etc.	Urinary retention with bladder balloon
Radiodermatitis	
Postradiotherapy or chemotherapy neuralgia	
Headache	
Vomiting	
Mucositis	
Proctitis	
Colitis	
Cystitis	

parents can err, for their psychological and sentimental involvement. In neonatal age in particular, but throughout the whole pediatric life span, it is important to use scales that give the level of basic pain, and not just the pain experienced in response to a sudden stimulus such as a heel-prick. So, scales developed uniquely for the assessment of acute procedural pain, such as PIPP (Preterm Infant Pain Profile) or DAN (Douleur Aigue du Nouveau-Né) [5] are of scarce utility for practical use; in fact, the aim of pain assessment is not knowing if an injection is painful, but assessing the base state of the patient [6]. These scales for acute procedural pain, on the converse, are useful for research purposes.

The Pain and Discomfort Scale (PADS) is used to assess pain in individuals without the cognitive capacity to assess internal experiences. It is a substitute of an expressed language. This instrument relies on facial expressions and body movements as indicators of acute pain and discomfort; it was designed to aid healthcare professionals to recognize, diagnose, and treat pain in patients with severe and profound communication difficulties [7, 8].

Clinical rating scales such as the FLACC (Face, Legs, Activity, Cry, Consolability) scale (Table 16.2) can be used in patients under 2 years of age [10].

Particularly useful scales for newborns are the CRIES (Crying, Requires oxygen, Increased vital signs, Expression, Sleep) scale or the EDIN (Echelle de la Douleur et Incomfort du Nouveau-né) scale (Fig. 16.1).

16.1 Pain Assessment

Table 16.2 FLACC scale

Criteria[9]	Score 0	Score 1	Score 2
Face	No particular expression or smile	Occasional grimace or frown, withdrawn, uninterested	Frequent to constant quivering chin, clenched jaw
Legs	Normal position or relaxed	Uneasy, restless, tense	Kicking or legs drawn up
Activity	Lying quietly, normal position, moves easily	Squirming, shifting, back and forth, tense	Arched, rigid or jerking
Cry	No cry (awake or asleep)	Moans or whimpers; occasional complaint	Crying steadily, screams or sobs, frequent complaints
Consolability	Content, relaxed	Reassured by occasional touching, hugging, or being talked to, distractible	Difficult to console or comfort

The final score is given by the sum of the single items

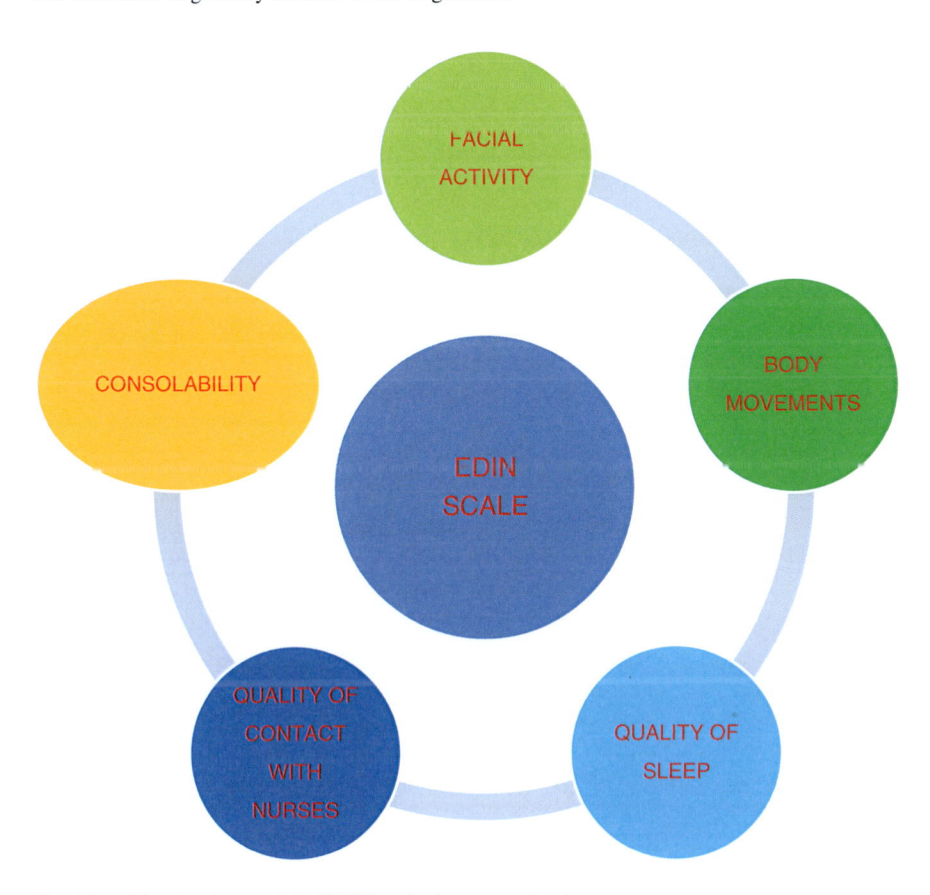

Fig. 16.1 The five items of the EDIN scale for neonatal pain

16.2 Sedation

Maintaining the consciousness of patients, even if they have minimal interaction with the environment, is essential and should be guaranteed as long as symptoms can be controlled. It is important to assess the sedation, in order to obtain the level of consciousness that is useful to the patient in that moment [11]. Several scales assess the sedation of a patient (see Table 16.3), for instance the Ramsay scale, the Richmond Agitation–Sedation Scale (RASS), or the Observer's Assessment of Alertness/Sedation (OAA/S) scale [12]. Sedative drugs are not analgesics, so before sedating patients, in any circumstance, make sure that the patients do not have pain and, if they have, treat it: sedation blunts the body response to pain, while it does not reduce pain itself. This is the reason why seldom we see an association of sedative drugs with painkillers. Consider sedating patients when they are so agitated that they can compromise their well-being and treatments or a thorough diagnosis (see Sect. 16.3). But do not only sedate patients to resolve their pain.

16.3 Refractory Symptoms

Refractory symptoms are clinical situations in which the patient's condition cannot be controlled without compromising their level of consciousness, despite having applied all the appropriate and proportional treatments. Refractory symptoms are not just difficult symptoms to treat and require the participation of various professionals as well as the use of specific techniques for their control [9, 13]. Pain, dyspnea, persistent emesis, and agitated delirium are the refractory symptoms most commonly requiring sedation [14].

It is important to assess if they have treatable causes, in order to assess if sedation is necessary or not, because sedating a patient can be necessary, but contextually the

Table 16.3 The Richmond Agitation–Sedation Scale

Score	Term	Description
+4	Combative	Overtly combative or violent; immediate danger to staff
+3	Very agitated	Pulls on or removes tube(s) or catheter(s) or has aggressive behavior toward staff
+2	Agitated	Frequent nonpurposeful movement or patient–ventilator dyssynchrony
+1	Restless	Anxious or apprehensive but movements not aggressive or vigorous
0	Alert and calm	Spontaneously pays attention to caregiver
−1	Drowsy	Not fully alert, but has sustained (more than 10 s) awakening, with eye contact, to voice
−2	Light sedation	Briefly (less than 10 s) awakens with eye contact to voice
−3	Moderate sedation	Any movement (but no eye contact) to voice
−4	Deep sedation	No response to voice, but any movement to physical stimulation
−5	Unarousable	No response to voice or physical stimulation

cause of their anxiety and stress should be found out and, if possible, removed. For example: (1) in a patient diagnosed with severe hypoxic-ischemic encephalopathy with delirium, a possible fluid and electrolyte disorder secondary to dehydration should be ruled out; (2) in a patient with a tumor that causes superior vena cava syndrome or nerve root compression, it is important to assess if palliative radiotherapy can be helpful; (3) in a patient with neurological disease with irritability, it is important to rule out the presence of a bladder balloon; (4) in a patient with severe cerebral palsy, spasticity and significant scoliosis, a possible fecal impaction or a need for an increase in muscle relaxants must be assessed; (5) always consider a possible withdrawal crisis from baclofen or tizanidine [15]. Palliative sedation can be overused [14] but if used properly, it is safe and does not lead to death [16]; anyway, it is important that all the aspects of the disease are considered and removed when possible, before proceeding toward a further and deeper step of sedative treatment.

References

1. Jobski K, Luque Ramos A, Albrecht K, Hoffmann F. Pain, depressive symptoms and medication in German patients with rheumatoid arthritis-results from the linking patient-reported outcomes with claims data for health services research in rheumatology (PROCLAIR) study. Pharmacoepidemiol Drug Saf. 2017;26(7):766–74. https://doi.org/10.1002/pds.4202. Epub 2017 Mar 26
2. Van den Beuken-van Everdingen MH, de Rijke JM, Kessels AG, Schouten HC, van Kleef M, Patijn J. Prevalence of pain in patients with cancer: a systematic review of the past 40 years. Ann Oncol. 2007;18(9):1437–49.
3. Neufeld NJ, Elnahal SM, Alvarez RH. Cancer pain: a review of epidemiology, clinical quality and value impact. Future Oncol. 2017;13(9):833–41.
4. Borsook D. Neurological diseases and pain. Brain. 2012;135(Pt 2):320–44. https://doi.org/10.1093/brain/awr271. Epub 2011 Nov 8
5. Maxwell LG, Fraga MV, Malavolta CP. Assessment of pain in the Newborn: an update. Clin Perinatol. 2019;46(4):693–707.
6. Bellieni CV. The limitations of pain scales. JAMA Pediatr. 2020;174(6):623. https://doi.org/10.1001/jamapediatrics.2020.0076.
7. Bodfish JW, Harper VN, Deacon JR, Symons FJ. Identifying and measuring pain in persons with developmental disabilities: a manual for the Pain and Discomfort Scale (PADS). Western Carolina Center Research Reports. 2001.
8. Phan A, Edwards CL, Robinson EL. The assessment of pain and discomfort in individuals with mental retardation. Res Dev Disabil. 2005;26(5):433–9. https://doi.org/10.1016/j.ridd.2004.10.001.
9. BC Center for Palliative Care. Refractory symptoms and palliative sedation. 2017. Accessed 5 May 2022. https://bc-cpc.ca/wpcontent/uploads/2019/06/17-RefractorySymptomsAndPalliativeSedationColourPrint.pdf.
10. Crellin DJ, Harrison D, Santamaria N, Babl FE. Systematic review of the face, legs, activity, cry and consolability scale for assessing pain in infants and children: is it reliable, valid, and feasible for use? Pain. 2015;156(11):2132–51. https://doi.org/10.1097/j.pain.0000000000000305.
11. Maltoni M, Scarpi E, Nanni O. Palliative sedation for intolerable suffering. Curr Opin Oncol. 2014;26(4):389–94. https://doi.org/10.1097/CCO.0000000000000097.

12. Lozano-Díaz D, Valdivielso Serna A, Garrido Palomo R, Arias-Arias Á, Tárraga López PJ, Martínez GA. Validation of the Ramsay scale for invasive procedures under deep sedation in pediatrics. Paediatr Anaesth. 2021; https://doi.org/10.1111/pan.14248. Epub ahead of print.
13. Garcia de Paso Mora M. Analgesia y sedación en Cuidados Paliativos Pediátricos. Bol Pediatr. 2013;53(224):68–73.
14. Stanford School of Medicine. Palliative care. Refractory symptoms. 2021. Accessed 5 May 2022. https://palliative.stanford.edu/palliative-sedation/definition-of-refractory-symptoms/
15. Suárez-Lledó A, Padullés A, Lozano T, Cobo-Sacristán S, Colls M, Jódar R. Management of tizanidine withdrawal syndrome: a case report. Clin Med Insights Case Rep. 2018;13(11):1179547618758022. https://doi.org/10.1177/1179547618758022.
16. Maltoni M, Pittureri C, Scarpi E, Piccinini L, Martini F, Turci P, Montanari L, Nanni O, Amadori D. Palliative sedation therapy does not hasten death: results from a prospective multicenter study. Ann Oncol. 2009;20(7):1163–9. https://doi.org/10.1093/annonc/mdp048.

Pharmacological and Non-Pharmacological Analgesia

17.1 Non-Pharmacological Analgesia

Non-pharmacological analgesic therapies include different types of interventions aimed to modify the environment and to activate endogenous strategies against pain. Research confirms the efficacy of non-pharmacological techniques for pediatric-neonatal treatment [1].

Anxiety and fear increase the pain experience [2], so the first approach to pain is creating a child-friendly environment where anxiety is reduced to minimum. A released hospital set is the prerequisite for many positive outcomes of our clinical activity.

Non-pharmacological methods are quite effective and are also popular among children for their fantastic and imaginative features; they are also not expensive and easily provided.

Pain relief through non-pharmacological analgesia occurs in two ways. The first is the production of endorphins, the second is the competitive inhibition of the stimulus. The production of endorphins occurs, for example, by using massage [3] or with the oral administration of sweet substances such as sugar or milk. Competitive inhibition occurs activating the inhibitory way descending from the cortex, which blocks the painful stimulus, for instance using distraction tools [4]; it also occurs through an inhibitory ascendent pathway, that closes a neural gate at the level of the spinal cord. In the latter case, interneurons present in the spinal cord, activated by tactile stimuli carried by the myelinated A fibers, block the painful stimuli carried by non-myelinated c fibers, through the so-called gate control of pain [5].

Cognitive and behavioral analgesic methods are used in older children. The main goal of cognitive methods is to divert attention from pain, selectively focusing it on different and more pleasant stimuli for the child [6]. The main goal of behavioral methods is to modify some emotional, behavioral, familiar, and situational factors that affect the child's response to pain. This will happen through relaxation with a series of techniques that provoke a sense of well-being [7].

Some examples of distraction and relaxation techniques

- Soap bubbles: it includes distraction from the formation of bubbles and relaxation in the exhalation necessary to produce and blow them.
- Magic glove: it simulates the child putting on an invisible glove, imagining it is massaging the hand in which the needle will be positioned, in order to desensitize it from pain.
- Breathing: it helps the child to reduce anxiety as early as the age of 3–4. This technique consists in inviting to make a deep breath, inflating the lungs, feeling the air coming in and out, and leading to an increasingly slower and deeper breathing. This technique captures the child's attention, reduces muscle tension, relaxes the diaphragm, and increases the oxygenation of the body.
- Visualization: (mental journey to a favorite place) is a complex cognitive-behavioral technique, with a hypnotic character, which consists in the use of the imagination, so that the child focuses on the mental image of a pleasant experience rather than on pain. In visualization, the child first invited to relax, then they are guided to imagine a situation and/or a favorite place in which they would like to be or where they have already been.
- Sensorial saturation: it is particularly effective in newborns and babies. It consists in the so-called 3Ts rule: touch (massage), talk (speaking softly), taste (giving oral sugar or milk). This can be obtained through breastfeeding or giving oral sugar with a syringe or on the pacifier while massaging and talking to the baby. The effect will appear as soon as the baby starts sucking rhythmically [8].
- Switch technique: it consists in focusing the child's attention on their own body and, in particular, on the "switches" that control the pain messages. After the child has reached a good level of concentration, through relaxation, he is invited to visualize a switch in his mind that can decrease the sensitivity to pain in the skin area where the procedure will have to be done; finally, they are explained that this switch can be lowered slowly (from 5, to 4, to 3, and so on up to 0) in order to make that specific area of the body less sensitive. After the procedure, it is essential to guide the child to remove the switch.
- Skin-to-skin contact: this has an important value in these processes: hugs, caresses, and holding hands. They have the property of inducing calm and sedation, in particular in newborns and toddlers

17.1.1 Rhythmic Patterns

Some of the above techniques are based on the activation of rhythmic patterns (Fig. 17.1). Rhythmic patterns are known to induce relaxation and to activate brain centers in the thalamus and amygdala [9] to get a sort of self-soothing. Our organism has several ways of self-soothing; among these, some are activated by rhythmic behaviors. Some rhythmic behaviors such as chewing, breathing, and walking [9, 10] are able to reduce anxiety and stress [11, 12]. The rhythmic nutritive or non-nutritive sucking performed by the neonate is a paradigm of this type of analgesic effect [13].

Fig. 17.1 The analgesic rhythmic patterns. Physiologic rhythmic pattern can induce relaxation and can be exploited to sooth the child. They also have an analgesic effect

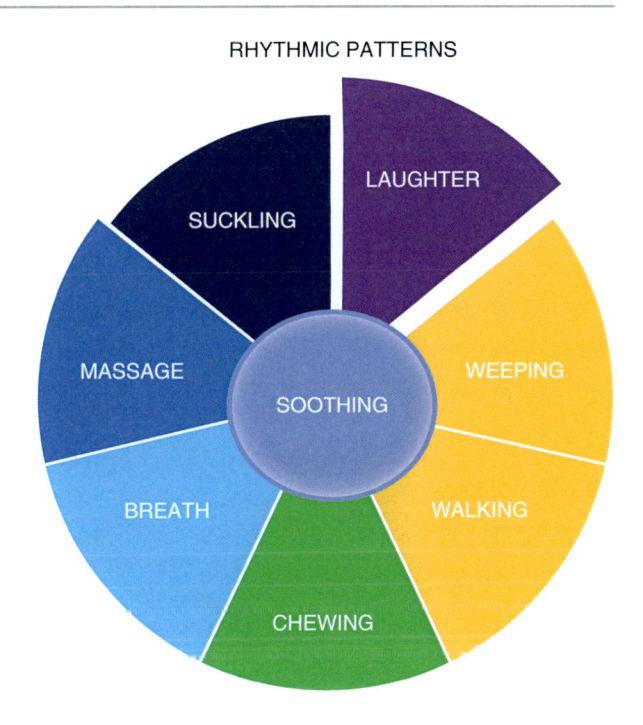

Of course, we should choose the appropriate non-pharmacologic treatment for the age and the peculiar features of the children we are treating. It depends on how much collaborative they are, and on the tasks they can accomplish. Neonates will have much benefit if they receive skin-to-skin contact during painful stimuli done for therapeutic reasons, if they smell their mother's odor, if they receive oral sugar [14]. Non-nutritive sucking acts on the behavior by exerting a calming effect, reducing heart rate and metabolic expenditure, and raising the pain threshold. It is another example of how much rhythmic behaviors induce relaxation and antagonize pain. The well-known "sensorial saturation" [15] is based on these principles: through the simultaneous administration of oral sweet solutions, massage, and vocal stimuli, it generates a distraction and at the same time a production of endorphins and a gate block. Sensorial saturation (Fig. 17.2) is used, for example, in the newborn and infant during painful stimuli, whose effects it cancels much more than the simple administration of oral sugar [16]. To sooth the toddler and obtain analgesic effect, it will be necessary to provide a gentle talk, massage, oral sugar, while for the older child different strategies will be appropriate: puppets, soap balls, telling stories. In the adolescence, it will be preferred talking about favorite places, watching television, magic glove, visualization, involvement, and music. All these strategies have the purpose of mainly modifying and altering the sensory dimension of pain, blocking the transmission of the painful stimuli along the peripheral and central nerve pathways, modifying the reception of nerve impulses or activating internal pain suppression mechanisms.

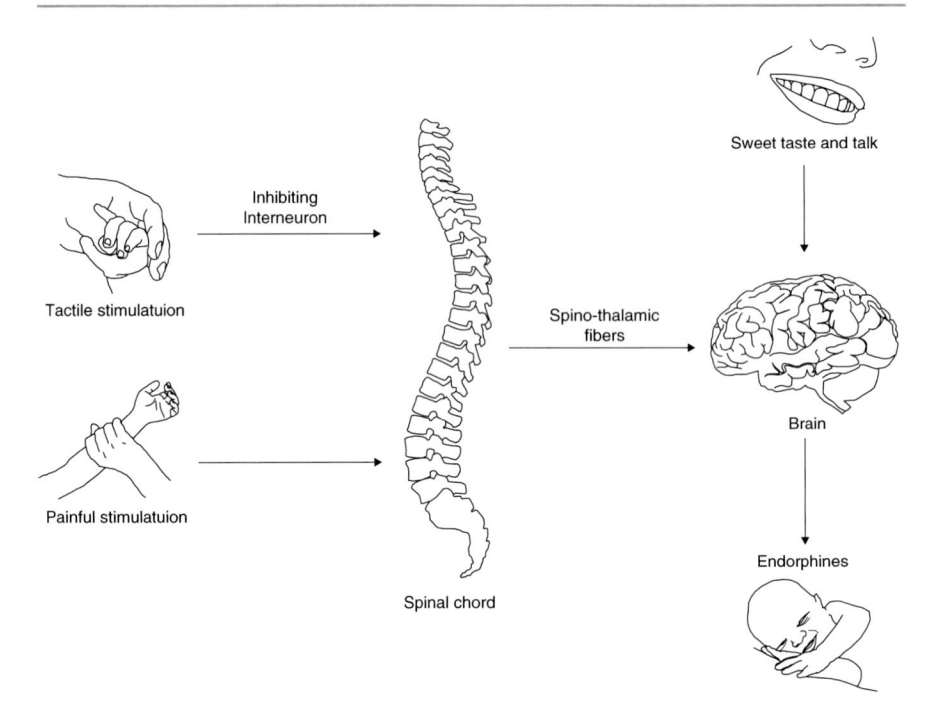

Fig. 17.2 Sensorial saturation. Sensorial saturation exploits the effect of three types of stimulations: touch, that activates the gate control at the level of the spinal cord; talk and taste that stimulate the descending inhibitory pathways (Courtesy of Carlo V. Bellieni © 2016 CV Bellieni)

These approaches are not automatically analgesic, but they need a gentle approach, preferably by a caregiver whom children have acquaintance and confidence with. The environment is crucial: in an overcrowded and noisy room, the positive effect of these strategies will be annihilated.

Do not forget the importance of ice therapy. This is mostly indicated in the management of pain from inflammation after trauma. There are many possibilities for this intervention: blocks of ice, sprays, gloves filled with water and ice or with frozen water. Avoid using ice as a painkiller in the newborn.

17.2 Opioids and Other Analgesics

17.2.1 The Earliest Steps of Pharmacological Analgesia

Pain treatments for pediatric palliative care rely on the same basis as those for adults. It is a four-step scale (Fig. 17.3), at whose base is the treatment with nonsteroidal analgesic drugs and acetaminophen; if pain is not controlled at the first step, we pass to the second, that is the treatment with mild opioids such as codeine or tramadol, to pass then, if necessary, to the third stage, namely strong opioids (morphine, fentanyl). The extreme stage is neural surgery or radiotherapy.

17.2 Opioids and Other Analgesics

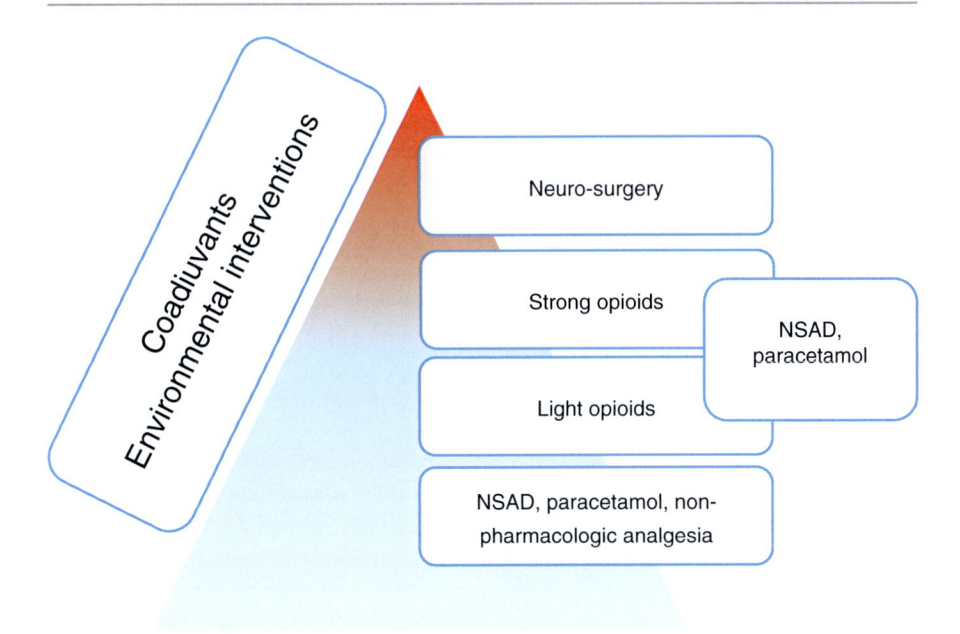

Fig. 17.3 Pharmacologic therapy for acute pain. When pain soars, more active drugs or treatments should be used. Consider always the availability of coadiuvants, the interventions on the environment, and the psychological support

The use of non-steroidal analgesics should be done carefully, for the possible evenience of collateral consequences in the case of excessive dosing; nonetheless, this should not retain us from their use: pain should always be avoided in any patient, in particular in those who are experiencing a tragic and terminal disease.

Dexmedetomidine—often administered via intranasal—is a relatively new drug approved at the end of 1999 by the Food and Drug Administration for humans use for short-term sedation and analgesia (<24 h) in the intensive care unit. Dexmedetomidine is a useful sedative agent with analgesic properties, hemodynamic stability, and which lets the patients recover respiratory function in those mechanically ventilated, facilitating early weaning [17]. Intranasal dexmedetomidine is a potentially useful medication for procedural sedation and in the management of complex wound dressings during palliative care. It provides short-term sedation, anxiolysis, and analgesia [18].

Another promising drug is a derivate of the chili pepper: *capsaicin*. Capsaicin is a molecule used in clinical trials as an experimental stimulus to evoke pain; nonetheless, awareness also grew that capsaicin was a powerful analgesic, and that it also leads to focal degeneration of nociceptors. Few studies on its use in children are available [19]. Highly concentrated topical capsaicin was approved to treat postherpetic neuralgia and, in Europe, other neuropathic pain conditions [20]. In focal pain conditions, there is appreciation that capsaicin may be given by injection to knockout nociceptors and achieve pain control. The major impediment to the clinical use of capsaicin is the immediate sense of burning. However, despite the high dosing associated with topical use, pain is quite circumscribed, lasting in the order of minutes to hours in exchange for months of therapeutic benefit [21].

17.2.2 Opioids and Opiates

Poppy-derived drugs, as all analgesics, have an interesting story (Fig. 17.4). Opiates have long been known as natural substances, found in the juice of the seeds of the poppy or *Papaver somniferum*. Its dry, fermented juice is called opium and contains a mixture of opiate alkaloids. In 1806, the German chemist Friedrich Serturner managed to isolate the main element of opium in its pure form, which he called morphine [22]. After minimal chemical alterations, it was possible to obtain semi-synthetic opiates. Now, it is possible to obtain completely synthetic opioids, almost without chemical relation with morphine, but with the same effect.

The term opiate is often used instead of opioid. However, the term opiates refers to the origin of the substance: they are substances that are extracted from the capsule of the poppy plant. By extension, also morphine-derived chemicals are referred to this way. The term opioid is used to designate those endogenous or exogenous substances that have an effect similar to that of morphine and possess intrinsic activity. Not all opiates are opioids, and not all opioids are opiates.

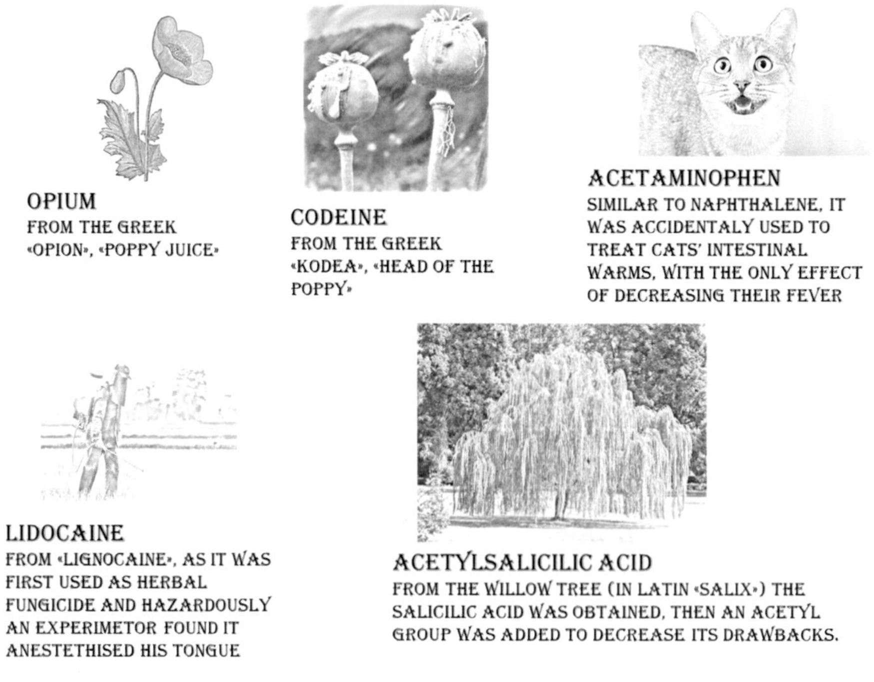

OPIUM
FROM THE GREEK
«OPION», «POPPY JUICE»

CODEINE
FROM THE GREEK
«KODEA», «HEAD OF THE POPPY»

ACETAMINOPHEN
SIMILAR TO NAPHTHALENE, IT WAS ACCIDENTALY USED TO TREAT CATS' INTESTINAL WARMS, WITH THE ONLY EFFECT OF DECREASING THEIR FEVER

LIDOCAINE
FROM «LIGNOCAINE», AS IT WAS FIRST USED AS HERBAL FUNGICIDE AND HAZARDOUSLY AN EXPERIMETOR FOUND IT ANESTETHISED HIS TONGUE

ACETYLSALICILIC ACID
FROM THE WILLOW TREE (IN LATIN «SALIX») THE SALICILIC ACID WAS OBTAINED, THEN AN ACETYL GROUP WAS ADDED TO DECREASE ITS DRAWBACKS.

Fig. 17.4 Pills of history of the most known analgesic drugs

There are currently no exhaustive guidelines on the use of opioids for analgesia in the pediatric population. The Centers for Disease Control and Prevention [23] opioid prescribing guide for chronic pain indicates that there is limited evidence for the use of opioids for children and adolescents. Therefore, pediatric practices have been adapted according to the experiences of the adult population [24].

Patient-controlled analgesia pumps have revolutionized the field of pain management. They are electronic programmable devices which can be tailored with respect to patient's requirements: the patient can activate the pump according to the level of pain they are experiencing. They can be used in pediatrics [25].

17.2.3 Main Opioids Used in Pediatrics

There are several commercially available opioids, but not all are appropriate for the pediatric population. Fentanyl, morphine, and methadone are opioids used by all ages, including newborns. Oxycodone and hydromorphone are labeled by the US Food and Drug Administration for use in children older than 6 months of age [26, 27]. Hydrocodone is used off label for patients under 2 years of age [27, 28]. The American Pain Society and the Institute for Safe Medication Practices do not recommend meperidine for pediatric analgesic use, due to the accumulation of a toxic metabolite (normeperidine) that can cause central nervous system toxicity, including seizures [29]. This effect is especially significant in patients with renal dysfunction. The US Food and Drug Administration issued a risk warning for codeine and tramadol in children under 12 years of age and limited use in children 12–18 years of age due to respiratory and even fatal risks [30]. Oxymorphone is not routinely recommended for use in pediatric patients, as it carries a black box warning of respiratory depression and other warnings regarding high risk of addiction, abuse, misuse, overdose, and death [26, 27].

Concerns about opioid use in the pediatric population also rise from the current opioid epidemic in the United States, and consequent recommendations have been issued for storage (Table 17.1) and prescription (Table 17.2).

In 2016, the Centers for Disease Control and Prevention (CDC) issued new guidelines for prescribing opioids [32]. They recommend that doctors avoid prescribing benzodiazepines concurrently with opioids whenever possible. Both prescription opioids and benzodiazepines now carry FDA "black box" warnings on their labels highlighting the dangers of using these drugs together [33].

17.3 Adjuvant Drugs

Adjuvant drugs are used to strengthen the effectiveness of analgesics, treating concomitant pain aggravating symptoms, and providing independent analgesia for specific types of pain; they can be used at all stages of the analgesic scale (Fig. 17.4). Of course, several of these drugs are not intended for little children or babies and should be selected with caution [34].

Table 17.1 Recommendations for patients for safe opioid use, storage, and disposal from ref. Reddy et al. [31]

Safe use	Safe storage	Safe disposal
Only use medications prescribed for you by your medical provider	Store your pain medication in a safe place that is not visible to others besides yourself or a designated caregiver who helps manage your medicines	Use take-back programs in law enforcement offices, hospitals, and pharmacies in your community
Do not share pain medications with others	Place pain medications under lock and key	Visit the drug enforcement administration web site to look for the next prescription drug take Back in your area
Only take medications as prescribed	Store pain medications away from young children, adolescents, and pets	Do not share or give unused pain medications to anyone
Call your medical provider if pain is not controlled, and do not change the dosage yourself	Do not tell others that you are taking pain medications	Mix unused medication with undesirable material, such as cat litter and discard in a sealed container
Do not stop taking pain medications without talking to your medical provider	Keep track of the number of medicines you have used. Report any missed medicine to law enforcement authorities	Some medications may be flushed in the toilet if other disposal options are not readily available
Do not take alcohol and other illicit drugs when taking pain medications		
Give your medical provider a complete list of medications you take		

17.3.1 Steroids

Steroids are among the most commonly used adjuvant medicines for the management of several types of cancer pain: metastatic bone pain, neuropathic pain, and visceral pain [35]. Corticosteroids have mainly anti-inflammatory activity and by reducing the edema of the nervous structures they have an analgesic effect. Dexamethasone or prednisone can be added to opioids for the treatment of pain in brachial or lumbosacral plexopathy. Undesirable effects of prolonged corticosteroid therapy can be myopathy, hyperglycemia, weight gain, and dysphoria.

17.3.2 Anticonvulsants

Cancer-related neuropathic pain is common and can be caused by the disease or by cancer treatment, and anticonvulsants are commonly used as adjuvant medications for the treatment of neuropathic pain. Some antiepileptics have been reported to be effective for the treatment of neuropathic pain (see [36]); these include gabapentin,

17.3 Adjuvant Drugs

Table 17.2 The CDC recommendations for opioid prescription in adults

1.	Non-pharmacologic therapy and nonopioid pharmacologic therapy are preferred for chronic pain. Clinicians should consider opioid therapy only if expected benefits for both pain and function are anticipated to outweigh risks to the patient. If opioids are used, they should be combined with non-pharmacologic therapy and nonopioid pharmacologic therapy, as appropriate
2.	Before starting opioid therapy for chronic pain, clinicians should establish treatment goals with all patients, including realistic goals for pain and function, and should consider how opioid therapy will be discontinued if benefits do not outweigh risks. Clinicians should continue opioid therapy only if there is clinically meaningful improvement in pain and function that outweighs risks to patient safety
3.	Before starting and periodically during opioid therapy, clinicians should discuss with patients known risks and realistic benefits of opioid therapy and patient and clinician responsibilities for managing therapy
4.	When starting opioid therapy for chronic pain, clinicians should prescribe immediate-release opioids instead of extended-release/long-acting (ER/LA) opioids
5.	When opioids are started, clinicians should prescribe the lowest effective dosage. Clinicians should use caution when prescribing opioids at any dosage, should carefully reassess evidence of individual benefits and risks when considering increasing dosage to $\geq$50 morphine milligram equivalents (MME)/day and should avoid increasing dosage to $\geq$90 MME/day or carefully justify a decision to titrate dosage to $\geq$90 MME/day
6.	Long-term opioid use often begins with treatment of acute pain. When opioids are used for acute pain, clinicians should prescribe the lowest effective dose of immediate-release opioids and should prescribe no greater quantity than needed for the expected duration of pain severe enough to require opioids. Three days or less will often be sufficient; more than 7 days will rarely be needed
7.	Clinicians should evaluate benefits and harms with patients within 1–4 weeks of starting opioid therapy for chronic pain or of dose escalation. Clinicians should evaluate benefits and harms of continued therapy with patients every 3 months or more frequently. If benefits do not outweigh harms of continued opioid therapy, clinicians should optimize other therapies and work with patients to taper opioids to lower dosages or to taper and discontinue opioids
8.	Before starting and periodically during continuation of opioid therapy, clinicians should evaluate risk factors for opioid-related harms. Clinicians should incorporate into the management plan strategies to mitigate risk, including considering offering naloxone when factors that increase risk for opioid overdose, such as history of overdose, history of substance use disorder, higher opioid dosages ($\geq$50 MME/day), or concurrent benzodiazepine use, are present
9.	Clinicians should review the patient's history of controlled substance prescriptions using state prescription drug monitoring program (PDMP) data to determine whether the patient is receiving opioid dosages or dangerous combinations that put him or her at high risk for overdose. Clinicians should review PDMP data when starting opioid therapy for chronic pain and periodically during opioid therapy for chronic pain, ranging from every prescription to every 3 months
10.	When prescribing opioids for chronic pain, clinicians should use urine drug testing before starting opioid therapy and consider urine drug testing at least annually to assess for prescribed medications as well as other controlled prescription drugs and illicit drugs
11.	Clinicians should avoid prescribing opioid pain medication and benzodiazepines concurrently whenever possible
12.	Clinicians should offer or arrange evidence-based treatment (usually medication-assisted treatment with buprenorphine or methadone in combination with behavioral therapies) for patients with opioid use disorder

Here, we report the recommendations made by the CDC for the opioid prescription in adults (https://www.cdc.gov/drugoverdose/pdf/guidelines_factsheet-providers-a.pdf), from which usually children's indications are extrapolated pregabalin, carbamazepine, and valproate [37]. Anticonvulsants are indicated in neuropathic pain, especially if throbbing or burning. Phenytoin, carbamazepine, valproate, and clonazepam suppress spontaneous neuronal burning and are used to control pain that complicates nerve injury. Carbamazepine should be used with caution in cancer patients undergoing chemo-radiotherapy, due to the potential risk of transient suppression of myelopoietic function. As usual, the blood dosage of anticonvulsants should be monitored for the side effects they have. Gabapentin and pregabalin have a specific indication for neuropathic pain and have been identified for this disease as first choice drugs (along with amitriptyline) in a recent survey [38].

17.3.3 Antidepressants

Cancer-related neuropathic pain is common and can be caused by the disease or cancer treatment. Two classes of antidepressants, tricyclic antidepressants and selective serotonin and norepinephrine reuptake inhibitors, are commonly used as adjuvant medicines for the treatment of neuropathic pain [34]. The most used antidepressant in these cases is amitriptyline, but when taken with opioids, it often causes anticholinergic side effects which can be serious, particularly respiratory problems [39]. The analgesic effects appear within 2 weeks after starting therapy and are maximal after 4–6 weeks.

17.3.4 Neuroleptics

Among the antipsychotic drugs, only metotrimeprazine has a specific analgesic action, perhaps exerted through an α-adrenergic block; it is a valid alternative to opioids because it does not have their typical side effects. However, metotrimeprazine can cause sedation and hypotension so it must be administered with care. Hydroxyzine combines the analgesic effect with the anxiolytic and also antiemetic effect; therefore, it can be used to treat pain in anxious patients [40]. Metotrimeprazine, a well-known drug, can be administered in a variety of ways and can be an effective tool in the treatment of complicated end-of-life symptoms in children [41].

17.3.5 Bisphosphonates and Calcitonin

Bisphosphonates reduce bone pain because they inhibit the activity of osteoclasts and are useful in patients with bone metastases; therefore, they can reduce the need for analgesics [42]. They can be used intravenously and reduce bone pain in children and adolescents [43]. Calcitonin also acts like bisphosphonates and, as they do, it also reduces hypercalcemia from bone metastases. Calcitonin, in addition to relieving lower back pain in patients with osteoporosis, could also usefully act on neuropathic pain [44]. However, further confirmatory studies are needed for these drugs.

17.3.6 Placebo

The analgesic response to placebo is frequent and may be mediated by endogenous opioid pathways [45]. Placebo is effective in some patients for only a short period of time and should not be used in the treatment of cancer pain although its use is justified by the enormous psychological component of cancer pain.

17.3.7 Antineoplastic Drugs

Antineoplastic treatments such as chemotherapy, hormonal and biological therapies, radiotherapy are not used specifically to treat pain; however, they can induce analgesia if they cause a significant reduction in tumor mass.

17.3.8 The Conundrum of Cannabinoids

Cannabinoids, the chemical components of marijuana, can relieve nausea [46], anorexia and has also some effect on neuropathic pain [47, 48]. In pediatric cancer treatment, some analogs such as synthetic cannabinoids, or dronabinol, are routinely prescribed to manage nausea and anorexia [49, 50]. Cannabinoids may also have other potential effects although the evidence is limited to preclinical studies [51]. The American Academy of Pediatrics recognizes medical marijuana as a potential supportive measure for children with severe illness [52, 53]. With regard to pain, the International Association for the Study of Pain (IASP) nonetheless found "that there is a lack of sufficient evidence to endorse the general use of cannabinoids for the treatment of pain" [54]. Thence, Medical Marijuana has not been adopted in pediatrics for several reasons. First, there is concern about adverse psychiatric and cognitive effects in developing children [55]. Second, appropriate formulations and dosages are not known [56]. Third, critics cite concern that the access to Medical Marijuana may promote the illicit use or ingestion of toxic substances. Finally, marijuana is a Schedule 1 controlled substance, which means that there are no currently accepted medical claims and it has a high potential of abuse; Schedule 1 classification designates Medical Marijuana's acquisition, use, or recommendation as federal offenses [57, 58].

17.3.9 Off-Label Drugs

A useful list of off-label analgesic drugs available for children (Table 17.3) has recently been issued [59]. "In Italy, the off-label use is governed by Law 648/96 that has identified a list of medications with a therapeutic indication other than that authorized, used in clinical practice for consolidated use and data from scientific literature. These drugs, once inserted in the list of medicinal products established by Law 648/96, are administered under the physician's direct responsibility and can be

Table 17.3 Off-label analgesic drugs (from [59], modified)

Drug	On-label use	Off-label use
HYOSCINE BUTYLBROMIDE	Pill in children >14 years, supp in children >6 years: Spastic—Painful events of urinary and genital tract	1. Iv administration for intestinal obstruction due to peritonitis in pediatric patients with cancer
		2. Iv administration for reduction of secretions and rattle in terminally ill patient
DEXMEDETOMIDINE	Procedural analgo-sedation outside the operating room (not operating room Anesthesia—NORA) in children with difficult airway management and child with seizure disorders who must undergo diagnostic studies for locating epileptogenic foci	1. Control of stressful symptoms from disease or procedure and fix sleep outside the ICU in patients in palliative care, not responsive to conventional therapies
		2. Intranasal route of administration
	Analgo-sedation of critical infants and children in ICU, mechanically ventilated and poorly responsive to conventional analgo-sedation treatment.	
FENTANYL	Premedication for any type of anesthesia (also local) both in the postoperative period as during surgery	1. Transdermal, iv use for acute and/or chronic pain management from cancer and not, in children in PPC
		2. Transmucosal use for procedural/acute/breakthrough pain in PPC
GABAPENTIN	Pill in children >6 years: Adjunctive therapy in the treatment of partial seizures in the presence or absence of secondary generalization	Neuropathic or mixed pain in children older than 2 years in palliative care
	>12 years: Monotherapy in the treatment of partial seizures in the presence or absence of secondary generalization	
KETAMINE	Im, iv, and continuous infusion administering	1. Use in patients in PPC for managing procedural or mixed/neuropathic pain that does not respond to other therapy, alone or in combination/replacement for opioid analgesics
	Use for induction and maintenance of general anesthesia from neonatal and premedication in children older than 1 month	2. Intranasal administration

17.3 Adjuvant Drugs

Table 17.3 (continued)

Drug	On-label use	Off-label use
KETOROLAC	The safety and efficacy in children have not been established. The use of this drug is therefore contraindicated below 16 years	By mouth and sublingual use for children 4–15 years old, for a maximum period of 5 days, in patients receiving PPC without vascular access, for management of moderate/severe acute episodic nociceptive pain, which integrate other analgesia if not effective, in the course of pathology eligible to PPC or in terminal illness
	Pills and drops: Used to treat short-term (max 5 days) moderate postoperative pain	
	Iv/im: Indicated in the short-term treatment (maximum 2 days) for moderate-severe postoperative pain	
	By mouth/im use for treatment of acute pain starting from 16 years of life, iv from 6 months	
LIDOCAINE	Peripheral and regional anesthesia, surgical stomatology	1. Nebulized use for the treatment of cough refractory to other therapies, if pulmonary metastases
		2. Intravenous use to treat neuropathic pain in patients in PPC not responsive to conventional therapies
MIDAZOLAM	Iv: Conscious sedation before and during diagnostic or therapeutic procedures with or without local anesthesia; Anesthesia: Premedication before induction of anesthesia; sedation in ICU	1. Intranasal use for its low invasiveness and high speed of administration in the absence of venous access, in urgent cases in patients aged over 1 month in PPC
	Children 3 months–18 years: Treatment of acute prolonged seizures	2. Intravenous use to manage non-painful end-of-life distress symptoms
	Children >1 month: Treatment of status epilepticus or following crises	
ONDANSETRON	Pills, syrup, vials in children ≥6 months to control chemotherapy-induced nausea and vomiting	Control of nausea and vomiting during opioid therapy in patients aged >6 months in palliative care
	Vials in children ≥1 month for prevention and treatment of postoperative nausea and vomiting	
SCOPOLAMINE	Not marketed in Italy	Treatment of hypersalivation in patients in palliative care and end of life via transdermal

Iv in vein, *Im* intramuscular, *PPC* Pediatric palliative care reimbursed by the National Health Service" [59]. Recently, ketamine has showed good results in promoting analgesia and sedation in pediatric palliative care settings [60].

17.4 Sedation

Sedatives are not strictly analgesic drugs, but can cooperate with them as adjuvants, when pain has become a refractory symptom, that is when it is necessary to lower the patient's level of opposition to make analgesic drugs effective. Sedation is the reduction of the level of consciousness with the aim of reducing or abolishing the cognitive capacity in a patient [61]. The most important goal of sedation is to calm and placate the patient. Sedation can be classified in many ways, based on its depth, reversibility, duration, etc.

Three objectives of sedation can be distinguished into: (1) Minimal sedation: decreasing the level of consciousness during a painful and shocking procedure; (2) Moderate sedation: to lower the level of consciousness as needed and the time it takes the patient to control a symptom at a given time; (3) Deep sedation: to reduce the level of consciousness of a patient with advanced and terminal illness. In cases of minimal and moderate sedation, drugs with a shorter half-life are usually used such as: midazolam, propofol [62], nitrous oxide [63] and also—although not a sedative drug—transmucosal or inhalation fentanyl can be used, which produces analgesia and a decrease in the level of consciousness. Dexmedetomidine is a highly selective α2-adrenergic receptor agonist of the new generation which is associated with sedative effects and sparing of analgesics, reduction of delirium and agitation, perioperative sympatholysis, cardiovascular stabilizing effects, and preservation of respiratory function; it can be administered intranasally [64]. In case of deep sedation, continuous infusions of drugs are usually necessary, for example, midazolam [65] and in case of delirium Levomepromazine. The consequences resulting from sedation in each of the groups are different: in group 1, there is a punctual and reversible decrease in consciousness; sedation in group 2 is usually longer, and in group 3 the depth is determined by achieving the symptom control: its duration depends on the evolution of the disease and its depth may be reduced if the symptom is under control.

Sedation performed in pediatric palliative care units is not intended to accelerate the end-of-life process [66]. Allowing a natural death is one of the goals of pediatric palliative care: once a symptom has been controlled and the desired depth of sedation is achieved, it is not recommended to increase the sedation, as long as the patient is calm and asymptomatic. The ideal sedation in the agony phase is that which allows the patient to have moments of wakefulness while being asymptomatic. Maria Nabal, editor of the journal Medicina Paliativa, wrote that "If, in our hedonistic society, professionals and family project our suffering onto the patient, we can be tempted to sedate in a somewhat indiscriminate way. In an attempt to safeguard what we mistakenly understand as charity, we free the patient from his autonomy" [67].

It is essential to know if there is symptom control and then to determine if sedation can be reversed at some point. For example: [29] in a patient with a convulsive state we can administer a continuous subcutaneous infusion of midazolam, which can be reduced and stopped if that state ceases; [52] acute bleeding in a patient with leukemia may require deep acute sedation, due to the great distress it generates, and if the bleeding is controlled the subsequent sedation can be stopped.

References

1. Koizumi T, Kurosawa H. Survey of analgesia and sedation in pediatric intensive care units in Japan. Pediatr Int. 2020;62(5):535–41. https://doi.org/10.1111/ped.14139.
2. Cimpean A, David D. The mechanisms of pain tolerance and pain-related anxiety in acute pain. Health Psychol Open. 2019;6(2):2055102919865161. https://doi.org/10.1177/2055102919865161.
3. Day JA, Mason RR, Chesrown SE. Effect of massage on serum level of beta-endorphin and beta-lipotropin in healthy adults. Phys Ther. 1987;67(6):926–30. https://doi.org/10.1093/ptj/67.6.926.
4. Melzack R. From the gate to the neuromatrix. Pain. 1999;(Suppl 6):S121–6. https://doi.org/10.1016/S0304-3959(99)00145-1.
5. Melzack R, Wall PD. Pain mechanisms: a new theory. Science. 1965;150(3699):971–9. https://doi.org/10.1126/science.150.3699.971.
6. Campbell CM, Witmer K, Simango M, Carteret A, Loggia ML, Campbell JN, Haythornthwaite JA, Edwards RR. Catastrophizing delays the analgesic effect of distraction. Pain. 2010;149(2):202–7. https://doi.org/10.1016/j.pain.2009.11.012. Epub 2010 Feb 25.
7. Argoff CE, Albrecht P, Irving G, Rice F. Multimodal analgesia for chronic pain: rationale and future directions. Pain Med. 2009;10(Suppl 2):S53–66. https://doi.org/10.1111/j.1526-4637.2009.00669.x.
8. Bellieni CV, Cordelli DM, Marchi S, Ceccarelli S, Perrone S, Maffei M, Buonocore G. Sensorial saturation for neonatal analgesia. Clin J Pain. 2007;23(3):219–21.
9. Sasaguri K, Yamada K, Yamamoto T. Uncovering the neural circuitry involved in the stress-attenuation effects of chewing. Jpn Dent Sci Rev. 2018;54(3):118-126. doi: https://doi.org/10.1016/j.jdsr.2018.03.002. Epub 2018 Apr 6.
10. Raad G, Tanios J, Azoury J, Daher A, Fakih C, Bakos HW. Neurophysiology of cognitive behavioural therapy, deep breathing and progressive muscle relaxation used in conjunction with ART treatments: a narrative review. Hum Reprod Update. 2021;27(2):324–38. https://doi.org/10.1093/humupd/dmaa048.
11. Goldbeck F, Xie YL, Hautzinger M, Fallgatter AJ, Sudeck G, Ehlis AC. Relaxation or regulation: the acute effect of mind-body exercise on heart rate variability and subjective state in experienced Qi Gong Practitioners. Evid Based Complement Alternat Med. 2021;2021:6673190. https://doi.org/10.1155/2021/6673190.
12. Mofleh R, Kocsis B. Delta-range coupling between prefrontal cortex and hippocampus supported by respiratory rhythmic input from the olfactory bulb in freely behaving rats. Sci Rep. 2021;11(1):8100. https://doi.org/10.1038/s41598-021-87562-8.
13. Uematsu H, Sobue I. Effect of music (Brahms lullaby) and non-nutritive sucking on heel lance in preterm infants: a randomized controlled crossover trial. Paediatr Child Health. 2019;24(1):e33-e39. doi: https://doi.org/10.1093/pch/pxy072. Epub 2018 Jul 24. Erratum in: Paediatr Child Health. 2019;24(1):63.
14. Bucsea O, Pillai RR. Non-pharmacological pain management in the neonatal intensive care unit: managing neonatal pain without drugs. Semin Fetal Neonatal Med. 2019;24(4):101017. https://doi.org/10.1016/j.siny.2019.05.009. Epub 2019 Jun 5. Erratum in: Semin Fetal Neonatal Med. 2021;26(2):101027.

15. Bellieni CV, Tei M, Coccina F, Buonocore G. Sensorial saturation for infants' pain. J Matern Fetal Neonatal Med. 2012;25(Suppl 1):79–81. https://doi.org/10.3109/14767058.2012.663548. Epub 2012 Mar 7
16. Locatelli C, Bellieni CV. Sensorial saturation and neonatal pain: a review. J Matern Fetal Neonatal Med. 2018;31(23):3209-3213. doi: https://doi.org/10.1080/14767058.2017.1366983. Epub 2017 Aug 23.
17. Takrouri MS, Seraj MA, Channa AB, el-Dawlatly AA, Thallage A, Riad W, et al. Dexmedetomidine in intensive care unit: a study of hemodynamic changes. Middle East J Anesthesiol. 2002;16:587–595.
18. Ferguson L, Wilson M. Intranasal dexmedetomidine: procedural sedation in palliative care: a case report. Palliat Med. 2021;3:2692163211022184. https://doi.org/10.1177/02692163211022184. Epub ahead of print
19. Goncalves D, Rebelo V, Barbosa P, Gomes A. 8% Capsaicin patch in treatment of peripheral neuropathic pain. Pain Physician. 2020;23(5):E541–8.
20. European Medicine Agency. Qutenza product information. Annex 1: Summary of product characteristics. 2015. Accessed 5 May 2022. http://www.ema.europa.eu/docs/en_GB/document_library/EPAR_Product_Information/human/000909/WC500040453.pdf.
21. Chung MK, Campbell JN. Use of capsaicin to treat pain: mechanistic and therapeutic considerations. Pharmaceuticals (Basel). 2016;9(4):66. https://doi.org/10.3390/ph9040066.
22. Schmitz R. Friedrich Wilhelm Sertürner and the discovery of morphine. Pharm Hist. 1985;27(2):61–74.
23. CDC. Guidelines for prescribing opioids for chronic pain. 2016. Accessed 5 May 2022. https://www.cdc.gov/drugoverdose/pdf/Guidelines_At-A-Glance-508.pdf.
24. Schechter NL, Walco GA. The potential impact on children of the CDC Guideline for prescribing opioids for chronic pain: above all, do no harm. AMA Pediatr. 2016;170(5):425–6.
25. Hatef J, Smith LGF, Veneziano GC, Martin DP, Bhalla T, Leonard JR. Postoperative pain protocol in children after selective dorsal rhizotomy. Pediatr Neurosurg. 2020;55(4):181–7. https://doi.org/10.1159/000509333. Epub 2020 Sep 7
26. Lexicomp Online. Pediatric and neonatal Lexi-drugs online. Hudson, OH: Wolters Kluwer Clinical Drug Information Inc; 2019. Accessed 19 Jan 2019.
27. Matson KL, Johnson PN, Tran V, Horton ER, Sterner-Allison J; Advocacy Committee on behalf of Pediatric Pharmacy Advocacy Group. Opioid use in children. J Pediatr Pharmacol Ther. 2019;24(1):72-75. doi: https://doi.org/10.5863/1551-6776-24.1.72.
28. Verghese ST, Hannallah RS. Acute pain management in children. J Pain Res. 2010;3:105–23.
29. American Academy of Pediatrics, Committee on Psychosocial Aspects of Child and Family Health, American Pain Society, Task Force on Pain in Infants, Children, and Adolescents. The assessment and management of acute pain in infants, children, and adolescents. Pediatrics. 2001;108(3):793–7.
30. Jin J. Risks of codeine and tramadol in children. JAMA. 2017;318(15):1514.
31. Reddy A, de la Cruz M. Safe opioid use, storage, and disposal strategies in cancer pain management. Oncologist. 2019;24(11):1410-1415. doi: https://doi.org/10.1634/theoncologist.2019-0242. Epub 2019 May 16.
32. Dowell D, Haegerich TM, Chou R. CDC guideline for prescribing opioids for chronic pain — United States, 2016. MMWR Recomm Rep. 2016;65 https://doi.org/10.15585/mmwr.rr6501e1er.
33. National Institute for Drug Abuse. Benzodiazepines and opioids. 2021. Accessed 5 May 2022. https://www.drugabuse.gov/drug-topics/opioids/benzodiazepines-opioids.
34. WHO. Guidelines for the pharmacological and radiotherapeutic management of cancer pain in adults and adolescents. Geneva: World Health Organization; 2018.
35. Bruera E, Watanabe S. Corticosteroids as adjuvant analgesics. J Pain Symptom Manag. 1994;9(7):442–5.
36. Fallon MT. Neuropathic pain in cancer. Br J Anaesth. 2013;111:105–11.

37. Dosenovic S, Jelicic Kadic A, Miljanovic M, Biocic M, Boric K, Cavar M, Markovina N, Vucic K, Puljak L. Interventions for Neuropathic Pain: An Overview of Systematic Reviews. Anesth Analg. 2017;125(2):643–52.
38. de Leeuw TG, der Zanden TV, Ravera S, Felisi M, Bonifazi D, Tibboel D, Ceci A, Kaguelidou F, de Wildt SN; On Behalf Of The Gapp Consortium. Diagnosis and treatment of chronic neuropathic and mixed pain in children and adolescents: results of a survey study amongst practitioners. Children (Basel). 2020;7(11):208. doi: https://doi.org/10.3390/children7110208.
39. NHS-UK. Amitriptyline for pain and migraine. 2021. Accessed 5 May 2022. https://www.nhs.uk/medicines/amitriptyline-for-pain/.
40. Mimick M. Postoperative analgesia—comparison of methotrimeprazine (nozinan®) and meperidine (demerol®) as postoperative analgesia agents. Can Anaesth Soc J. 1972;19:87–96.
41. Hohl CM, Stenekes S, Harlos MS, Shepherd E, McClement S, Chochinov HM. Methotrimeprazine for the management of end-of-life symptoms in infants and children. J Palliat Care. 2013;29(3):178–85.
42. Hoskin PJ. Bisphosphonates and radiation therapy for palliation of metastatic bone disease. Cancer Treat Rev. 2003;29(4):321–7.
43. Celin MR, Simon JC, Krzak JJ, Fial AV, Kruger KM, Smith PA, Harris GF. Do bisphosphonates alleviate pain in children? A systematic review Curr Osteoporos Rep. 2020;18(5):486-504. doi: 10https://doi.org/10.1007/s11914-020-00621-3. Erratum in: Curr Osteoporos Rep. 2020 Oct 29.
44. Ito A, Yoshimura M. Mechanisms of the analgesic effect of calcitonin on chronic pain by alteration of receptor or channel expression. Mol Pain. 2017;13:1744806917720316. https://doi.org/10.1177/1744806917720316.
45. Zubieta JK, Bueller JA, Jackson LR, Scott DJ, Xu Y, Koeppe RA, Nichols TE, Stohler CS. Placebo effects mediated by endogenous opioid activity on mu-opioid receptors. J Neurosci. 2005;25(34):7754–62. https://doi.org/10.1523/JNEUROSCI.0439-05.2005.
46. Sallan SE, Zinberg NE, Frei E III. Antiemetic effect of delta-9tetrahydrocannabinol in patients receiving cancer chemotherapy. N Engl J Med. 1975;293(16):795–7.
47. de Jong FA, Engels FK, Mathijssen RH, et al. Medicinal cannabis in oncology practice: still a bridge too far? J Clin Oncol. 2005;23(13):2886–91.
48. Kogan NM, Mechoulam R. Cannabinoids in health and disease. Dialogues Clin Neurosci. 2007;9(4):413–30.
49. Ananth P, Ma C, Al-Sayegh H, Kroon L, Klein V, Wharton C, Hallez E, Braun I, Michelson K, Rosenberg AR, London W, Wolfe J. Provider perspectives on use of medical marijuana in children with cancer. Pediatrics. 2018;141(1):e20170559. https://doi.org/10.1542/peds.2017-0559. Epub 2017 Dec 12
50. Elder JJ, Knoderer HM. Characterization of dronabinol usage in a pediatric oncology population. J Pediatr Pharmacol Ther. 2015;20(6):462–7.
51. Velasco G, Hernández-Tiedra S, Dávila D, Lorente M. The use of cannabinoids as anticancer agents. Prog Neuropsychopharmacol Biol Psychiatry. 2016;64:259–66.
52. American Academy of Pediatrics, Committee on Substance Abuse; Committee on Adolescence. The impact of marijuana policies on youth: clinical, research, and legal update. Pediatrics. 2015;135(3):584–7.
53. Ammerman S, Ryan S, Adelman WP; Committee on Substance Abuse Committee on Adolescence. The impact of marijuana policies on youth: clinical, research, and legal update. Pediatrics. 2015;135(3):e769–85.
54. IASP. IASP position statement on the use of cannabinoids to treat pain 2021. Accessed 5 May 2022. https://www.iasp-pain.org/publications/iasp-news/iasp-position-statement-on-the-use-of-cannabinoids-to-treat-pain/.
55. Levy S. Effects of marijuana policy on children and adolescents. JAMA Pediatr. 2013;167(7):600–2.
56. Nierengarten MB. Guidelines needed for medical use of marijuana. Lancet Oncol. 2007;8(11):965.
57. Annas GJ. Medical marijuana, physicians, and state law. N Engl J Med. 2014;371(11):983–5.

58. Wang GS, Le Lait MC, Deakyne SJ, Bronstein AC, Bajaj L, Roosevelt G. Unintentional pediatric exposures to marijuana in Colorado, 2009–2015. JAMA Pediatr. 2016;170(9):e160971.
59. De Zen L, Marchetti F, Barbi E, Benini F. Off-label drugs use in pediatric palliative care. Ital J Pediatr. 2018;44(1):144. https://doi.org/10.1186/s13052-018-0584-8.
60. Benini F, Congedi S, Giacomelli L, Papa S, Shah A, Milani G. Refractory symptoms in paediatric palliative care: can ketamine help? Drugs Context. 2021;10:2021-2-5.
61. Krauss B, Green SM. Procedural sedation and analgesia in children. Lancet. 2006;367(9512):766–80. https://doi.org/10.1016/S0140-6736(06)68230-5.
62. Symington L, Thakore S. A review of the use of propofol for procedural sedation in the emergency department. Emerg Med J. 2006;23(2):89–93. https://doi.org/10.1136/emj.2005.023713.
63. Mohan R, Asir VD, Shanmugapriyan, Ebenezr V, Dakir A, Balakrishnan, Jacob J. Nitrousoxide as a conscious sedative in minor oral surgical procedure. J Pharm Bioallied Sci. 2015;7(Suppl 1):S248–50. https://doi.org/10.4103/0975-7406.155939.
64. Kaur M, Singh PM. Current role of dexmedetomidine in clinical anesthesia and intensive care. Anesth Essays Res. 2011;5(2):128–33. https://doi.org/10.4103/0259-1162.94750.
65. Heijltjes MT, Morita T, Mori M, Heckel M, Klein C, Stiel S, Miccinesi G, Deliens L, Robijn L, Stone P, Sykes N, Hui D, Krishna L, van Delden JJM, van der Heide A, Rietjens JA. Physicians' opinion and practice with the continuous use of sedatives in the last days of life. J Pain Symptom Manage. 2021;63(1):78–87. https://doi.org/10.1016/j.jpainsymman.2021.07.012. Epub ahead of print
66. Olsen ML, Swetz KM, Mueller PS. Ethical decision making with end-of-life care: palliative sedation and withholding or withdrawing life-sustaining treatments. Mayo Clin Proc. 2010;85(10):949-954. doi: https://doi.org/10.4065/mcp.2010.0201. Epub 2010 Aug 30.
67. Nabal M in Ethics and Sedation at the Closing of Life. Fundacion Victor Grifols I Lucas. 2003. Accessed 5 May 2022. https://www.fundaciogrifols.org/documents/4662337/4689043/monograph9.pdf/dc61f1db-1cb6-4d61-8f87-197fd9558c4b.

Psychological Approach 18

The family of the child in pediatric palliative care should also consider positively receiving help by a psychological professional, who will address them to the best intervention they are needing. It is important they do not consider themselves beyond any risk of depression or anxiety; this is true for both parents and the child. Depending on depressive symptoms, antidepressant use in patient undergoing palliative care ranges from 7% to 37% and over-the-counter drug use varies between 30% and 59% [1]. Psychological interventions for physical symptoms, such as fatigue, pain, dyspnea, and insomnia are available in pediatric palliative care units. Regarding psychological aspects, current reviews show small to large effects in the reduction of depression and anxiety symptoms through cognitive behavioral-based interventions, mindfulness-based interventions, and meaning-based interventions [2]. Meaning-based or dignity-based approaches were also used for improving mental and existential distress. These approaches, as well as the interventions on the environment to make it more child-friendly, implement and improve the effect of analgesic drugs and treatments (Fig. 18.1). Of course, we should never disdain the importance of psychotherapy, when needed.

18.1 Meaning-Based Approach

The meaning-making approach invites individuals to build a system of orienting beliefs, self-narratives, personal constructs, world assumptions, or schemas about their identity and the world [3]. This orienting system fosters a sense of meaning regarding the daily events individuals experience and their evolving life [4, 5]. The therapists attempt to "detoxify death" by having a direct discussion on death anxiety and fears.

Also, therapists provide an "existential nudge" which includes the creation of a sort of personal legacy [6]; this project focuses on whatever is most meaningful to

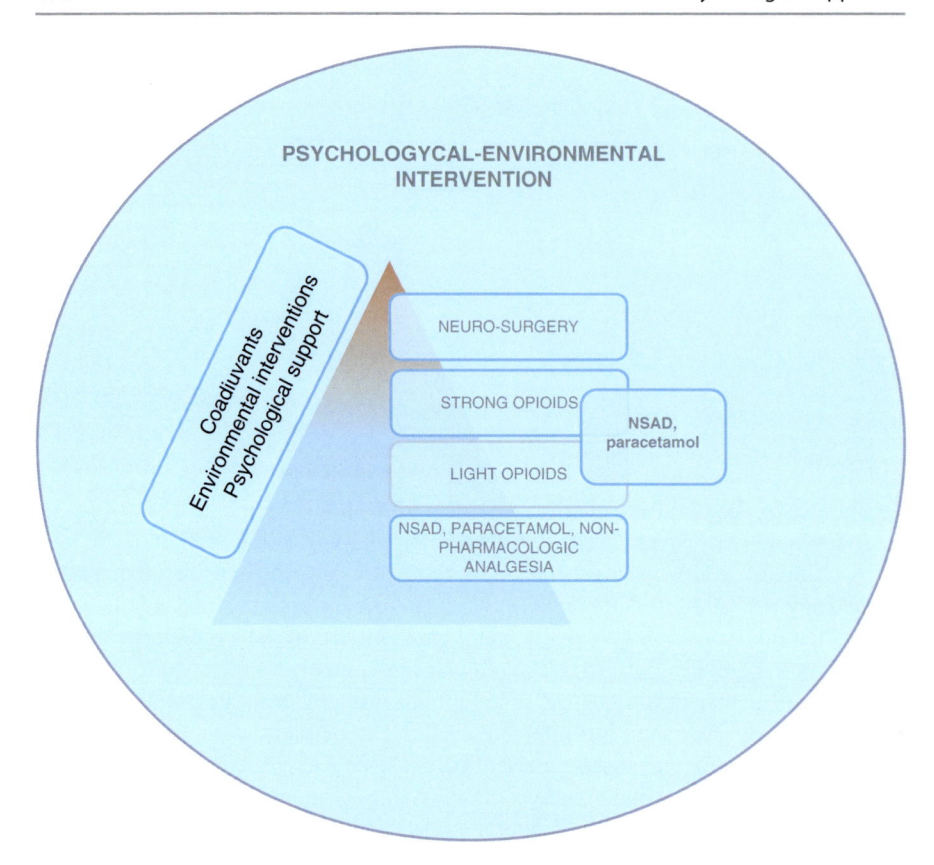

Fig. 18.1 Analgesic treatments framed in the psychological-environmental strategies. Without psychological-environmental strategies, the mere pain drugs are only partially effective

the patients and may feature mending fractured relationships, providing community service, traveling to places of interest, or finding ways to capture their life story (e.g., creating scrapbooks, videos, photo albums).

If the child is struggling with the uncertain nature of life following a sudden news about their health, getting meaning might entail a sense of valuing their life [7]. This therapy involves eight sessions when performed in a group, and seven sessions when performed individually. This therapy is typically facilitated by psychiatrists, psychologists, or psychology doctoral students and contains both didactic and experiential activities [8].

18.2 Dignity-Based Approach

Dignity therapy derives from the meaning-based approach. This psychotherapy protocol begins giving to the patient nine standard questions which are an opportunity for the patients' consideration and reflection about what they want to say. The questions will guide a conversation with a trained healthcare professional. Patients are given the questions before starting the session, in order to familiarize themselves with the possibilities this approach provides in terms of dealing with topics they may wish to discuss. The session is recorded, transcribed, and edited, after which a final file is produced and given to the patient [9, 10]. There is evidence that, with proper training, this form of treatment could be administered by professionals with skills and experience in psychosocial oncology. Healthcare professionals should also note the importance of using each clinical meeting as an opportunity to recognize, reinforce and, where possible, reaffirm the personality of the patients under their care [11]. Recent studies have investigated if this approach can be administered by nurses in palliative care set, but with disappointing results [12].

18.3 Promoting Resilience in Stress Management

Another means of improving children's response to a terminal diagnosis is PRISM (Promoting Resilience in Stress Management) technique. It is taught in person at the bedside and has four evidence-based skill-building sessions: stress management, goal-setting, positive reframing, and meaning-making. The one-on-one sessions are typically held every other week, and each session is taught by a trained interventionist [13, 14]. Abby Rosenberg, the ideator of this technique, sees PRISM as a targeted approach that helps "normalize the hard" [15]. "We are developing standardized and systematic ways to promote patient and family resilience in the setting of serious illness," she says. "Health is determined not only by biomedical processes, but also by emotions, behaviors and social relationships. If patients and families need certain resilience skills to thrive—and have better health outcomes because of those skills—we want to make sure they get that training. Our goal is to help them learn how to change their appraisal of difficult situations in real time and have greater quality of life in the future" [15].

18.4 Mindfulness

This word means awareness but with a particular meaning. It is not easy to describe it in words because it refers first of all to direct experience. Among the possible descriptions, that of Jon Kabat-Zinn, one of the pioneers of this approach, has become "classic" [16]. "Mindfulness means paying attention: a) with intention, b) at the present moment, c) in a non-judgmental way." It can also be described as a way to cultivate a fuller presence in the experience of the moment, in the "here and now."

In fact, the mindfulness approach derives from and is based on mindfulness meditation—one of the main meditative traditions of classical Buddhism—and consists precisely in proposing an introductory, initial level of meditation practice that is adequate and suitable for everyday contexts, to the normal life experience. In summary, an approach that can help patients put themselves in a different relationship with the discomfort they are experiencing. It is not a relaxation technique, and it is not a way to go into some form of trance, nor to clear the mind and reach "emptiness." It is not a way to guarantee an easy psychophysical well-being, some kind of "emotional spa," or is not a form of "doing good" that pushes us to accept everything, to accept uncritically what happens to us, and to be passive in the name of "acceptance."

Mindfulness has its positive effects even on children and adolescents [17]. It has been applied successfully in palliative care treatments [18]. It is not surprising that the primary applications have been in the clinical area: the 30-year pioneering work of Jon Kabat-Zinn, professor of medicine at the University of Massachusetts, has had a huge following in both medicine and psychotherapy [19]. Recent studies have elucidated its effectiveness in easing chronic pain [20, 21].

References

1. Jobski K, Luque Ramos A, Albrecht K, Hoffmann F. Pain, depressive symptoms and medication in German patients with rheumatoid arthritis-results from the linking patient-reported outcomes with claims data for health services research in rheumatology (PROCLAIR) study. Pharmacoepidemiol Drug Saf. 2017;26(7):766–74.
2. von Blanckenburg P, Leppin N. Psychological interventions in palliative care. Curr Opin Psychiatry. 2018;31(5):389–95. https://doi.org/10.1097/YCO.0000000000000441.
3. Kurtz KJ, Silliman DC. Object understanding: investigating the path from percept to meaning. Acta Psychol. 2021;216:103307. https://doi.org/10.1016/j.actpsy.2021.103307. Epub 2021 Apr 21.
4. de Vries FE, Godthelp A, Spruit JR, Ruissen AM, Tesselaar MET, Boekhout AH. Coping with social consequences of disease-related symptoms in patients with a metastatic small intestinal neuroendocrine tumour: a qualitative study. J Neuroendocrinol. 2021;33(3):e12956. https://doi.org/10.1111/jne.12956.
5. Gillies J, Neimeyer RA, Milman E. The meaning of loss codebook: construction of a system for analyzing meanings made in bereavement. Death Stud. 2014;38(1–5):207–16. https://doi.org/10.1080/07481187.2013.829367. Epub 2013 Nov 11.
6. Thomas LP, Meier EA, Irwin SA. Meaning-centered psychotherapy: a form of psychotherapy for patients with cancer. Curr Psychiatry Rep. 2014;16(10):488. https://doi.org/10.1007/s11920-014-0488-2.
7. Milman E, Neimeyer RA, Fitzpatrick M, MacKinnon CJ, Muis KR, Cohen SR. Prolonged grief symptomatology following violent loss: the mediating role of meaning. Eur J Psychotraumatol. 2018;8(Suppl 6):1503522. https://doi.org/10.1080/20008198.2018.1503522.
8. Breitbart W, Applebaum A. Meaning-centered group psychotherapy. In: Watson M, Kissane DW, editors. Handbook of psychotherapy in cancer care. 1st ed. Oxford: Wiley; 2011.
9. Chochinov HM, Hack T, Hassard T, Kristjanson LJ, McClement S, Harlos M. Dignity therapy: a novel psychotherapeutic intervention for patients near the end of life. J Clin Oncol. 2005;23(24):5520–5.
10. Martínez M, Arantzamendi M, Belar A, Carrasco JM, Carvajal A, Rullán M, Centeno C. 'Dignity therapy', a promising intervention in palliative care: a comprehensive systematic literature review. Palliat Med. 2017;31(6):492–509. https://doi.org/10.1177/0269216316665562. Epub 2016 Aug 26.
11. Thompson GN, Chochinov HM. Dignity-based approaches in the care of terminally ill patients. Curr Opin Support Palliat Care. 2008;2(1):49–53.
12. Nunziante F, Tanzi S, Alquati S, Autelitano C, Bedeschi E, Bertocchi E, Dragani M, Simonazzi D, Turola E, Braglia L, Masini L, Di Leo S. Providing dignity therapy to patients with advanced

cancer: a feasibility study within the setting of a hospital palliative care unit. BMC Palliat Care. 2021;20(1):129. https://doi.org/10.1186/s12904-021-00821-3.
13. Fladeboe KM, O'Donnell MB, Barton KS, Bradford MC, Steineck A, Junkins CC, Yi-Frazier JP, Rosenberg AR. A novel combined resilience and advance care planning intervention for adolescents and young adults with advanced cancer: a feasibility and acceptability cohort study. Cancer. 2021;127(23):4504–11. https://doi.org/10.1002/cncr.33830.
14. Rosenberg AR, Bradford MC, McCauley E, Curtis JR, Wolfe J, Baker KS, Yi-Frazier JP. Promoting resilience in adolescents and young adults with cancer: results from the PRISM randomized controlled trial. Cancer. 2018;124(19):3909–17. https://doi.org/10.1002/cncr.31666. Epub 2018 Sep 19.
15. Seattle Children's. Seattle Children's webpage: promoting resilience; reducing stress. 2021. Accessed May 5th 2022. https://www.seattlechildrens.org/about/stories/promoting-resilience-reducing-stress/
16. Kabath-Zinn J. Wherever you go, there you are. mindfulness meditation in everyday life. New York: Hachette Books Eds; 1995.
17. Perry-Parrish C, Copeland-Linder N, Webb L, Sibinga EM. Mindfulness-based approaches for children and youth. Curr Probl Pediatr Adolesc Health Care. 2016;46(6):172–8.
18. Latorraca COC, Martimbianco ALC, Pachito DV, Pacheco RL, Riera R. Mindfulness for palliative care patients. Systematic review. Int J Clin Pract. 2017;71(12). doi: https://doi.org/10.1111/ijcp.13034. Epub 2017 Nov 6.
19. Ludwig DS, Kabat-Zinn J. Mindfulness in medicine. JAMA. 2008;300(11):1350–2. https://doi.org/10.1001/jama.300.11.1350.
20. Hanley AW, Gililland J, Garland EL. To be mindful of the breath or pain: comparing two brief preoperative mindfulness techniques for total joint arthroplasty patients. J Consult Clin Psychol. 2021;89(7):590–600. https://doi.org/10.1037/ccp0000657. Epub 2021 Jun 24.
21. Pardos-Gascón EM, Narambuena L, Leal-Costa C, Ramos-Morcillo AJ, Ruzafa-Martínez M, van-der Hofstadt Román CJ. Effects of mindfulness-based cognitive therapy for chronic pain: a multicenter study. Int J Environ Res Public Health. 2021;18(13):6951. doi: https://doi.org/10.3390/ijerph18136951.

Part VI

Palliative Care and Our Fears

Pediatric palliative care puts caregivers in contact with some aspects of their lives people often remove or do not want to see. These are scary meanderings that reveal the obscure aspects of our own personality. Therefore, taking care of a dying child scares most medical doctors and nurses, provoking real troubles. Here, we illustrate these problematic situations, pointing out that fear should not be the last word in somebody's life or disease; it is a gate we should cross. It is important to see why this sense of fear exists in most doctors and nurses, and why they hide it with cynicism or sentimentalism, two wrong reactions. Thus, we will discuss three paradoxes in children's care that scare us deeply. We also will deal with the fear of death, that common feeling that disrupts most doctors and nurses, and with the rituals that the families perform in the eve of their beloved ones' death.

Dear reader before approaching the new section of the book, please take a moment for yourself, sit back and let that sink in…

Intermezzo

The Environment on Pain Perception
Jacques Prévert: Page d'écriture
Two and two are four
four and four are eight
eight and eight are sixteen …
Repeat! says the teacher
Two and two are four
four and four are eight
eight and eight are sixteen.
But here is the lyre bird
passing in the sky
the child sees it
the child hears it

*the child calls him
Save me
play with me
bird!
So the bird comes down
and play with the child
Two and two are four ...
Repeat! says the teacher
and the child plays
and plays with it ...
Four and four are eight
eight and eight are sixteen
and sixteen and sixteen what are they?
They aren't anything sixteen and sixteen
and especially not thirty-two
anyway
they go away.
And the child hid the bird
in his desk
and all the children
hear its song
and all the children
hear its music
and eight and eight in turn go
and four and four and two and two
in turn leave the camp
and one and one are neither one nor two
one by one also go away
And the lyre bird is playing
and the child is singing
and the teacher shouts:
When are you done fooling around!*

*But all the other kids
listen to the music
and the classroom walls
quietly collapse.
And the windows become sand again
the ink becomes water
the desks become trees
the chalk becomes cliff
the pen becomes a bird again*

Children's Pain Scares us

19.1 Our Fears

So far, we have seen that these are the features that make pediatric palliative care so special. First, we do not have dedicated drugs—unlike for adults—and we also have to adapt them to the weight of the patient instead of giving a standard dose. Second, children's ability to interact with their caregivers is different from the adult: children express themselves, but using a language that adults do not know or have forgotten, though they once used it. Third, a different way of expression corresponds to each age, often using a non-verbal language, as some nomadic tribes do, making it necessary to use a translator. Fourth, the ability to understand and to grasp the news changes from one age to another, as well as the ability to decide; so much so that, as the child grows up, the obligation of sharing decisions with them grows as well.

But a further aspect makes children's palliative care so special: the child scares us.

Fear is a diffuse emotion humans and other beings feel when attacked, or when they feel threatened or jeopardized. It is an important and useful feeling that gives us the signal for retrieving strengths and starting up after the perception of a risk. Yet, fear can become excessive when it starts a loop: fear makes brain activate the hypothalamic-pituitary-adrenal axis that induces the production of cortisol and adrenalin, which at their turn induce changes in heart rhythm and blood pressure; these changes are perceived by the brain through the amygdala that interpret them as an assault, so that a new cycle of anxiety and fear starts without an apparent reason [1]. Thus, fear can be an ally or a foe, depending on how we manage it.

In the case of pediatric palliative care, fear emerges for two reasons:

- Watching children's illness and struggle for life induces anxiety and fear in the bystanders and in caregivers: it can be managed or can overshadow our rationality, provoking panic, phobias, or depression that are transmitted to the child, who in turn increases their state of panic, provoking more anxiety in the onlookers, and so on. We are afraid that we might not bear the pain we are announcing them.

- Children have that sort of inner and innate madness that challenges the principle of non-contradiction which is the basis of our supposed rationality: for a child, a bottle is not just a bottle, but also a telescope or a gun; silence is not just meditation, but also time spent with magic thoughts. We are not able to decode it, but we are also unconsciously afraid that their madness is contagious, that it might break our professionalism, objectivity, and our mental integrity.

The scare these two points provoke is a special and underestimated feature of pediatric palliative care. All this can be described by three paradoxes that well illustrate this fear.

19.2 The Three Fearful Paradoxes

19.2.1 Paradox of the Simultaneous Blooming and Dying

Children in palliative care flourish and die at the same time. The main feature of the child is being thriving, growing up; diseases destroy this growth. We cannot accept this, it is unbelievable to see a fine oak growing up and simultaneously shriveling, a daring skyscraper being built while swinged down; we'd wish to hide that truth. We hide it to ourselves, and we wish to hide it from the parents and from the child, because, as human beings, we are not able to accept the paradox of something that thrives and dies at the same time: it is deplorable, an injustice, a waste, something repulsive. And therefore we don't want to admit that our nature is exactly this: we all are secretly flourishing and dying. And watching the blossoming and death of a child reminds this to us, forces us to realize it. The real drama for us is not just about a child who dies, but about the awareness that we are dying step by step, and the children are the tragic image of what secretly is happening to us: in the flesh of those children who are dying, we see ourselves who are dying as well [2]. That is not all: it also reminds us that our own children, the flesh of our flesh, will also die. In few words, the death of a child is a red alert, forcing us to grasp and watch the reality of our death.

19.2.2 Irrational-Reason Paradox

The second paradox is what we may call "an irrational rationality." The child is not afraid of death, while we are. Both in adolescence and in infancy, for different neuroevolutive reasons, the child does not fear death: earlier, because they do not understand it; later on, because they do not admit it into their thoughts, they do not rationalize death. They do not rationalize many things: children are almost completely irrational, and someone has even measured the extent that separates them from a rational thought [3]. What scares a human more than dealing with an irrational human who reminds them their inner irrationality? We talk about death, we can even decide of censoring death, but children simply have another world in their minds, where death is not death, where life is not life. They have magic thoughts, an incomplete theory of minds and of counterfactual thinking [4]. Their world is made of invulnerability, of the present day as the only horizon. They live a social life, they play, they love in a way different than ours, showing that another way of approaching the world and people is possible; that our rationality - that sees a bottle only as a bottle, or that is scared by speed and by height - is just one of the possible ways of considering the reality. They point out how irrational is our rationality because our rationality believes that only one rationality is possible.

We think to be rational beings, and this reassures us. But it should not. A century of psychoanalytic studies [5] has revealed that our supposed reason is actually what external constraints (superego) and internal unconscious inputs (id) have dug into our ego; we think to make free choices, but we make the choices that our id and our superego force us to make [6, 7]. We think we are rational, but our reasoning is invariably affected by internal legacies and external pressures [8]: just reflect on the violent and subtle force of the massmedia advertising machine.

Seeing a child who instead lives not weighing the facts, but using other measures (coherence, obedience, imitation, as we saw earlier in this book) upsets us, and shows us another world, in which the Aristotelian reason and syllogisms are not the supreme court, in which the language of love or instinctual repulsion have more value.

19.2.3 Paradox of the Spectator's Shadow

In the famous Platonic cave [9], those who turn their backs towards the exit from where the light enters, see in front of them the shadows of those who pass outside the door, confusing them with the reality, believing that the shadows are the sole and unique reality. The sense of this myth is to notice that we often mix up shadows with the reality. We can adapt this old myth to our field: we know only a standard way of speaking and a single and standard use of reason—those of the adult—and we confuse them with the fair way of reasoning and speaking though often the reality is much more than what we see and imagine [10].

What the myth of the cave does not say, is that inevitably on the wall in front of us not only the shadows of those who pass outside the door stand out (and we mistake their shadows with their reality), but also our own shadows, (the spectators' shadows), that we confuse with our (my) reality. What does the fake shadow represent in our true life? It is the role we have, that we mix up with our actual self; we have a duty, a job, and we think: "that is me!"; but we are much more than our role. We confuse our routine with our own reality: we are not able to see and detect what our "real reality" is (Fig. 19.1). But our deepest reality will never be identified with a standard role, an "employee" (in the etymologic sense of being folded to the necessities of the firm). Being "employees" is being functional to protocols, being aligned to the letter of the contracts, wheels of a gear.

The child scares us also in this case, because their naivety discloses the falsehood hidden under our employee masks. Children and babies do not consider us for our

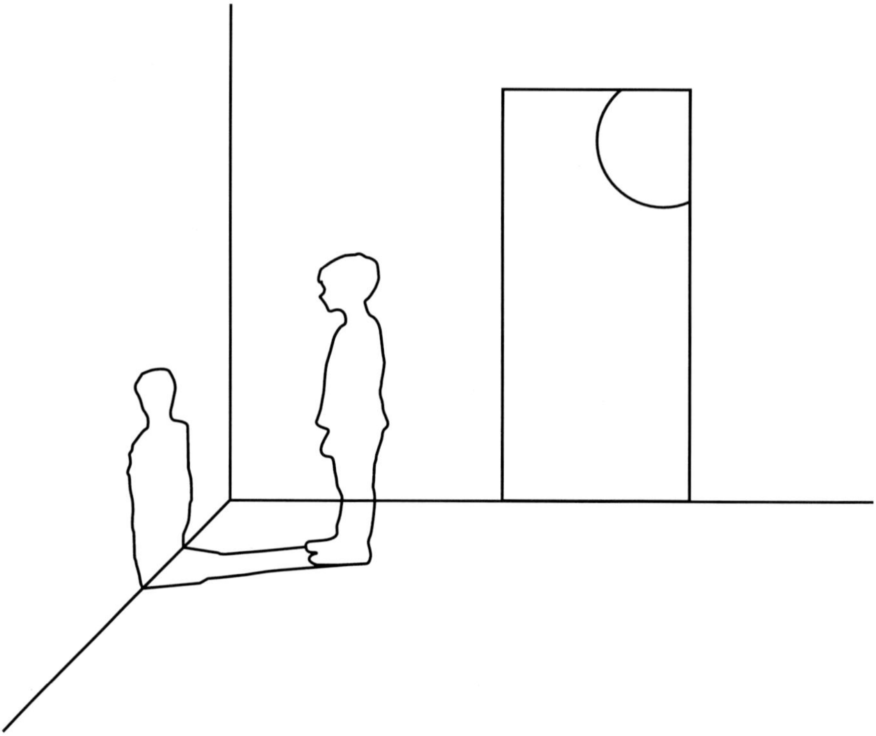

Fig. 19.1 The myth of the cave and the roles. In the myth of the cave, the spectators confused the shadows of external objects with the objects' themselves. Here, we argue that within the cave, we confuse our own shadows with our own reality. This means that we confuse our role (our shadow) with what we really are

role, but always for our commitment unto them and unto ourselves. As happens in the second part of the myth of the cave, when the spectators unveil the flaw, they watch the source of the life, the source of the light that has not yet been overwhelmed and disrupted by the barbarism of the world, by the madness of the id and the force of the superego.

Getting in touch with a child, learning how to get in touch with them scares us, but it is perhaps the path of the liberation for the adults. Heidegger said that thinking about death helps to become free from quackery and unauthenticity [11]. But also watching a child makes us free: death and birth are the two events that are not our property, that arrive without being planned and without being sought. We must look for this under the rubble, under the crust of mud of routine, of protocols, of what reduces people to their work. And watching how children behave, love or distrust helps.

References

1. Kozlowska K, Walker P, McLean L, Carrive P. Fear and the defense cascade: clinical implications and management. Harv Rev Psychiatry. 2015;23(4):263–87.
2. Jonas D, Scanlon C, Rusch R, Ito J, Joselow M. Bereavement After a Child's Death. Child Adolesc Psychiatr Clin N Am. 2018;27(4):579–90.
3. Bernard ME, Cronan F. The child and adolescent scale of irrationality: validation data and mental health correlates. J Cogn Psychother. 1999;13(2):121–32.
4. Nyhout A, Ganea PA. Scientific reasoning and counterfactual reasoning in development. Adv Child Dev Behav. 2021;61:223–53. https://doi.org/10.1016/bs.acdb.2021.04.005. Epub 2021 Jun 22
5. Freud S. The ego and the id (The standard edition of the complete psychological works of Sigmund Freud). The standard edition (17 September 1990). New York: W. W. Norton & Company; 1990.
6. Freud S. Introductory lectures on psychoanalysis. London: Penguin Books; 1991.
7. Wiesner JL. Mental freedom: who has control-the rider or the horse? Int J Dharma Stud. 2014;2:7.
8. Jacobs G: Limits to Rationality & the Boundaries of Perception. e-Journal of the World Academy of Art and Science. 2013;2(1):108–18.
9. Agrati LS: Plato's Myth of the Cave Images. A Didactic Analysis of the Mediation Function. Proceedings 2017;1(9):1091.
10. Ferguson AS. Plato's simile of light. Part II. The allegory of the cave. Class Q. 1922;16:15–28.
11. Glen L Sherman. Martin Heidegger's Concept of Authenticity: A Philosophical Contribution to Student Affairs Theory, Journal of College and Character. 2009,10.7.

Contagious Pains

20.1 Burnout

Another reason to be scared by children's pain exists: it is the subtle but real sense that their pain and suffering are contagious. This opens the door to an anguishing phenomenon: caregivers' burnout.

Burnout is a typical feature of most altruistic professions, such as nurses, firefighters, police, who should prevent disasters, but who in several cases fail, for destiny or for scarce resources, with consequent demotivation and grief. It is a progressive loss of idealism, energy, and motivation; it is frequent in health professionals. Herbert Freudenberg [1] coined the term burnout to define the signs and symptoms of a chronic exhausting syndrome, but it acquired its real importance from the investigations of Maslach [2]. The syndrome is characterized by a gradual deterioration of physical strength and tolerance under three aspects:

- Emotional fatigue: progressive loss of energy, mental wear-and-tear, and exhaustion.
- Depersonalization: the people you are dealing with are seen as objects or numbers.
- Negative feelings regarding professional fulfillment: pseudo-depressive manifestations and low self-esteem.

The professional burnout syndrome means feeling exhausted, demotivated, depressed, and overwhelmed by the suffering seen and by our sense of impotence. How could palliativists be exempted from this, living close to blooming lives that suddenly and irrevocably die? Most times caregivers prodigate their efforts in palliative care they know these efforts will be vane to save lives, the sentence of death having already been written. Of course, this is not completely true: their efforts bring release, calm, and a silent informal pleasure; but this is quite different from defeating a cancer or resuscitating a baby; only in few cases pediatric palliative care comes along with therapies aimed to resolve the base disease. In pediatric palliative care, anyone should face sorrow, and sorrow is something that grasps the soul.

The professional burnout syndrome has been studied from several perspectives [3]. In the psychosocial field, it is considered a process that consists of several stages that occur for the interaction of the personal characteristics of each individual with the stress of the work environment. In general, three types of causes can be identified: interpersonal, institutional, and those due to people's own characteristics. According to the EU "European Foundation for the Improvement of Living and Working Conditions" (https://www.eurofound.europa.eu/publications/report/2010/work-related-stress), in Europe, approximately 10% of workers suffer from depression, anxiety, or work stress, which is the second workers' health problem after back pain, and one of the main causes of absenteeism from work. Burnout is common in physicians who care for patients with serious illness, with rates greater than 60% in some studies [4]. Vitor Parola performed a review on the prevalence of burnout among palliative care professionals and concluded that "data revealed a prevalence of burnout of 17.3% among health professionals. Personal accomplishment was the sub-scale from the Maslach Burnout Inventory that had the most negative prevalence (19.5%). Nurses had higher levels of Emotional Exhaustion (19.5%) and Depersonalization (8.2%), and physicians had lower levels of Personal Accomplishment (41.2%). The prevalence of burnout was, however, higher in social workers (27%). The palliative care context with the highest prevalence of burnout was home care (19.6%)" [5].

Risk factors for burnout include working on small teams and/or in small organizations, working excessive hours and during the weekends, being younger than 50 years, excessive bureaucracy. Personal factors that can protect against burnout include mindfulness, exercise, healthy sleep patterns, avoiding substance abuse, and having adequate leisure time [4]. A study performed in Tampa, Florida, showed that 44% of the chiefs research officers registered a high degree of emotional exhaustion; the most mentioned factors were daily excess work and job dissatisfaction [6]. In the same year, the Finnish Institute for Occupational Health in Helsinki found out that burnout syndrome increases the risk of future absences among farm workers and of future occupational and non-occupational diseases [7]. Data from Mexico show that in Mexicali, Baja California, in 2004 a burnout prevalence of 44% was found among anesthesiologists, as well as among nurses [8]; and in Guadalajara the Regional Institute for Public Health Research identified 42.3% burnout affected workers among first-level care physicians who work in the metropolitan area [9].

Anyway, burnout must be prevented, and measured to intervene preventively. Scales to measure the personnel's level of burnout have been developed and are now available. One of the best known and used is the Maslach Burnout Inventory [10]. It is important that the hospitals organize burnout measurement, especially in the departments at higher risk, those in which one is more in contact with pain, suffering, and death. Ten years ago [11] we issued a charter of the rights of the child for a European scientific society, and the following point was included: "The prevention of stress for health workers is a right of the child." In fact, the prevention of burnout

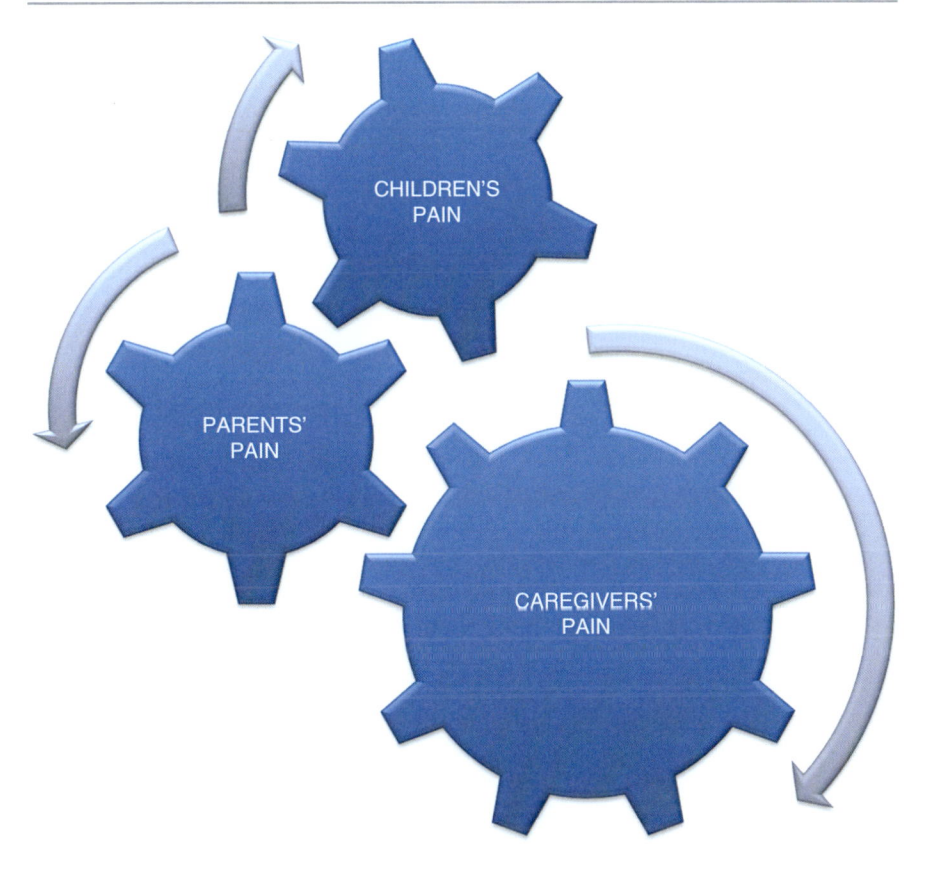

Fig. 20.1 Contagious pain. Parents, healthcare professionals, and children influence each other with their own pain

is not only a right of the worker, but of the patients themselves, because pain is contagious and a stressed doctor is less effective and performing than a relaxed one.

Pain and stress are contagious. Stressed parents infect their child with their stress; a stressed operator similarly infects the child with their stress (Fig. 20.1). But at the same time, parents and caregivers infect each other with their stress and the child absorbs and suffers this contagion, worsens, becomes depressed, and in turn sends the contagion back to the adults. It is a vicious cycle that soars indefinitely. We can call it the vortex of pain contagion [12]. That must stop, and we have the tools to do it.

20.2 Overcoming Burnout

Stress management programs range from relaxation to cognitive-behavioral treatments; patient-centered therapy has been found to be of utmost significance when it comes to preventing and treating burnout [13].

Mindfulness is one of these approaches. Mindfulness, that we have already dealt with in a previous chapter, is a self-directed practice for relaxing the body and calming the mind through focusing on present-moment awareness. The emphasis of mindfulness is staying in the present moment, with a non-judging, non-striving attitude of acceptance. Mindful meditation represents a complementary therapy that has been shown to be promising in the reduction of negative stress and the extraneous factors that lead to burnout. Many studies evaluated these "mindfulness-based" intervention, and showed that it plays an important role in decreasing stress and burnout [14]. Krasner and colleagues evaluated the effects of an intensive educational program that included mindful meditation, self-awareness exercises, narratives about clinical experiences, appreciative interviews, didactic material, and discussions on primary care physicians. Participants demonstrated improvements in awareness, which was correlated with an improvement in their overall mood, empathy (emotional exhaustion), personal accomplishment, and personality over the course period with sustained effects of up to 15 months [15].

Balint groups are a strategy for medical doctors to discuss their psychodynamics in relation to patients [16]. Michael Balint (1896–1970) tought to actively search the causes of anxiety and unhappiness and treat them, improving awareness rather than the direct suppression of symptoms [17]. A Balint group is a purposeful, regular meeting among physicians, with a trained facilitator or leader, to allow discussion of any topic that occupies a physician's mind outside of his or her usual clinical encounters, and to learn how to see the case from multiple perspectives (clinician's, patient's, and that of the relationships between them). The goal is to improve physicians' abilities to actively process their job, through a deeper understanding of how they are touched by the emotional impact of caring for certain patients [18]. Some studies have suggested that Balint sessions can have a promising positive effect in preventing burnout [19]. Balint exercises can reduce anxiety levels and exhaustion symptoms while improving the mental and physical well-being of healthcare workers.

Occupational interventions in the work settings can improve the emotional and work-induced exhaustion [20]. Combining both individual and organizational interventions can have a good impact in reducing burnout scores among physicians; therefore, multidisciplinary actions that include changes in work environmental risk factors, along with stress management programs that teach people how to cope better with stressful events, showed promising effects.

References

1. Freudenberg H. Burnout: the high cost of high achievement. Garden City, New York: Doubleday; 1980.
2. Maslach C. Burned-out. Can J Psychiatr Nurs. 1979;20(6):5–9.
3. Poghosyan L, Aiken LH, Sloane DM. Factor structure of the Maslach burnout inventory: an analysis of data from large scale cross-sectional surveys of nurses from eight countries. Int J Nurs Stud. 2009;46(7):894-902. doi: https://doi.org/10.1016/j.ijnurstu.2009.03.004. Epub 2009 Apr 10. Erratum in: Int J Nurs Stud. 2014;51(10):1416–7.

References

4. Horn DJ, Johnston CB. Burnout and self care for palliative care practitioners. Med Clin North Am. 2020;104(3):561-572. doi: https://doi.org/10.1016/j.mcna.2019.12.007. Epub 2020 Mar 2.
5. Parola V, Coelho A, Cardoso D, Sandgren A, Apóstolo J. Prevalence of burnout in health professionals working in palliative care: a systematic review. JBI Database System Rev Implement Rep. 2017;15(7):1905–33. https://doi.org/10.11124/JBISRIR-2016-003309.
6. Gwede CK, Johnson DJ, Roberts C, Cantor AB. Burnout in clinical research coordinators in the United States. Oncol Nurs Forum. 2005;32(6):1123.
7. Ahola K, Honkonen T, Virtanen M, Kivimäki M, Isometsä E, Aromaa A, Lönnqvist J. Interventions in relation to occupational burnout: the population-based health 2000 study. J Occup Environ Med. 2007;49(9):943–52.
8. Palmer LY, Prince R, Medina C, Figueroa M, López R, Rodríguez G. Prevalencia del síndrome de burnout en docentes de la Universidad autónoma de Baja California, Mexicali, México. Rev Cuba Salud Trabajo. 2016;17(3):36–40.
9. Aranda C, Pando M. Síndrome de burnout y apoyo social en los médicos familiares de base del Instituto Mexicano del Seguro Social (IMSS) Guadalajara, México. Rev Psich Fac Med Barc. 2004;31(4):196–205.
10. Maslach C, Jackson SE. The measurement of experienced burnout. J Occup Behav. 1981;2(2):99–113.
11. Guimaraes H, Sanchez-Luna M, Bellieni CV, Buonocore G; Union of European Neonatal and Perinatal Societies. Ethical charter of Union of European Neonatal and Perinatal Societies. J Matern Fetal Neonatal Med. 2011;24(6):855-858. doi: https://doi.org/10.3109/14767058.2010.531314. Epub 2010 Dec 1.
12. Wang H, Liu Y, Hu K, Zhang M, Du M, Huang H, Yue X. Healthcare workers' stress when caring for COVID-19 patients: an altruistic perspective. Nurs Ethics. 2020;27(7):1490-1500. doi: https://doi.org/10.1177/0969733020934146. Epub 2020 Jul 14.
13. Romani M, Ashkar K. Burnout among physicians. Libyan J Med. 2014;9:23556. https://doi.org/10.3402/ljm.v9.23556.
14. Goodman MJ, Schorling JB. A mindfulness course decreases burnout and improves well-being among healthcare providers. Int J Psychiatry Med. 2012;43:119–28.
15. Krasner M, Epstein RM, Beckman H, Suchman AL, Chapman B, Mooney CJ, et al. Association of an educational program in mindful communication with burnout, empathy, and attitudes among primary care physicians. JAMA. 2009;302:1284–93.
16. Gajree N. Can Balint groups fill a gap in medical curricula? Clin Teach. 2021;18(2):158-162. doi: https://doi.org/10.1111/tct.13298. Epub 2020 Oct 19.
17. Lustig M. Balint groups: an Australasian perspective for psychiatrists. Australas Psychiatry. 2016;24(1):30-33. doi: https://doi.org/10.1177/1039856215613013. Epub 2015 Nov 4.
18. Roberts M. Balint groups: a tool for personal and professional resilience. Can Fam Physician. 2012;58(3):245–7.
19. Kjeldmand D, Holmstrom I. Balint groups as a means to increase job satisfaction and prevent burnout among general practitioners. Ann Fam Med. 2008;6:138–45.
20. Awa W, Plaumann M, Walter U. Burnout prevention: a review of intervention programs. Patient Educ Couns. 2010;78:184–90.

The Fear of Death and the Errors It Provokes

21.1 How Fear Can Overshadow Our Judgment

We are concerned about how decisions on end of life are taken. It can happen that we dump our sense of guilt or our fear of pain on the patient, and transfer how we feel unto them. We can think they are feeling what we are feeling or what we desire them to feel [1]. The presence of children's pain makes us less objective and throw our empathy beyond its due limits. So that we see suffering where it is not present, or we deny to be seeing it because its sight is unbearable for us. The mere use of inference can lead to underestimate children's quality of life and to overrate their pain [2] because our brain reacts so to the vision of a potentially painful event in the others [3] and is subject to their own psychological state [4]. In a randomized trial, we saw that mothers rate their children's pain higher when they are trying to sooth them during a vein puncture, rather than when they are just watching the procedure, being in the same room [5].

This means that the common ways to judge a disease and in particular if a life is worth living are utterly influenced by our prejudices or by our optimism. But a more objective way is needed. Unfortunately, other people's pain and suffering makes us unbalanced. It is normal: maybe this is due to some shortcut that make us mirror the patient's status and pain, and in some of us it is terrible, so that we do not accept it, neither we want to see it [6].

If we do not want to see the pain, other criteria are used in end-of-life decisions, most tied to a utilitaristic approach. Here, I do not want to stigmatize this philosophic thought, but I am sure that human life is to be weighted with different tools than those used to decide on the decline of a factory or on the performance of a car. We should decide what the best interest of a patient is, if for them is preferable to go on living or not. But this is really hard. The problem is that not only it is difficult to say what the patient's best interest is, but it is also problematic to define what the word "interest" really means. The word interest has three meanings. The first is the economic meaning: "interest" is what you get from the loan of money to a bank. The term "interest" also means the attention that the subject voluntarily pays to a thing. Third, the word "interest" means advantage, utility. Here, we speak of interest as "advantage, utility"; however, the translation "advantage" is not exempt from some contaminations of the other two meanings when we talk, so that it cannot be separated from the *economic interest* or from the *patient's attention*. In short, we should consider the interest of the patients as the advantage they get from a treatment, but often we consider it according to how much money their treatments cost (economic interest) and if they have a state of consciousness to make them "interested" (patient's attention).

Patients' interest is also weighted on the future prognosis, made on the bases of the present scientific knowledges. This is correct, under the condition of being aware that what yesterday was considered intractable, tomorrow may be overcome. It is the case of several congenital disease, such as some heart defects or trisomies that now have a realistic possibility of survival [7, 8]. We will discuss this in the next paragraph.

What is the real benefit or advantage for a person? Who really knows? What we had thought to be an advantage, sometimes turned out to be a loss and vice versa. To understand the advantage of an action, you need two requisites: one retrospective (assessing if the desired goal has been achieved) and one prospective (considering the various options, disasters and possibilities that the new situation will bring). Unfortunately, the latter is out of the range of what we can foresee. In fact, we make projects, but the bad news about projects is that at most they come true: the end of a love an open a way towards a new one, more exciting, or the rejection at a university exam may unveil a new style of life [9]. Of course, in the case of extreme brain damages, the utility of the actions to cure them seems very unlikely, but not all brain damages are equal and not all have a devasting effect, and while many people with disabilities go into depression, some accept—after an often hard path—the new though tough life [10, 11].

We should also consider the problem of children's pain. Several cases of treatment withdrawal that have permitted babies to die have been reported by massmedia in the last few years [12]; unfortunately, we have never had notice of a careful measurement of the pain they were going through or of thorough prediction of the future events that wouold provoke pain to these babies. This could have been a useful weapon to decide if the baby was able to bear the ongoing treatments, and would have avoided many polemics. So, it seems that the baby's best interest been decided without an important element. Anyway, also using only the pain assessment to decide is a weak solution: if we decide that beyond a certain threshold the cures should be withdrawn (or continued if below that threshold), we behave partially, while pain should be one of several points to assess in deciding on end of life.

But the contact with the patient's pain makes us less objectives. Using those ways we have described -namely the best interest principle and the pain assessment- can help, but they have several limitations, and they cannot make us enter the deep secrets of an impaired child. And when pain is overwhelming, we can decide abruptly, or cynically, or without considering the current advances of the medical art.

21.2 Balancing Research and Respect

Sometimes we can shift too quickly to palliative care treatments and interrupt lifesaving treatments, as if there were no more hopes of healing. Anyway, as hinted above, some diseases that once were considered intractable, now have found important progress and hopes. Some examples are here due. It is the case of the hypoplastic left heart syndrome. A recent review [8] showed how its treatment shifted from mere palliative care to long-term survival. The management of hypoplastic left heart syndrome has changed substantially over the past four decades. In the 1970s, children with hypoplastic left heart syndrome could only receive supportive care, and most of these children died within the neonatal period. The advent of the Norwood procedure in the early 1980s has changed the prognosis for these children, and most of them now undergo a series of surgical treatments that can support survival beyond the neonatal period and into early adulthood.

It is also the case for trisomy 13 and 18 that are still considered two birth-defects that impose not to resuscitate the patient, and active treatments are denied in these cases. On the converse, some authors, after becoming aware of changes in outcomes, now recommend a case-by-case assessment of cardiac surgical interventions for children with trisomy 13 or 18 [7, 13]. Coordinated care planning and interdisciplinary communication are relevant in cardiac surgical considerations for children with these genetic conditions.

It is also the case of extremely preterm babies, who following several guidelines are not actively assisted at birth, but trying to give them a chance, their survival has now increased in a consistent rate [14], with respect to several years ago. Many advocate to change those guidelines as obsolete [15].

Is a sense of compassion in front to others' pain that leads us to be less proactive with these babies? Or is the respect unto their autonomy and the fear of treating them as a part of a clinical trial that will not benefit them (maybe it will benefit future babies) and that might prolong their sufferings? This problem is a challenge for all neonatologists and geneticists; it is worth reflecting.

References

1. Redelmeier DA, Dickinson VM. Determining whether a patient is feeling better: pitfalls from the science of human perception. J Gen Intern Med. 2011;26(8):900–6. https://doi.org/10.1007/s11606-011-1655-3. Epub 2011 Feb 19.
2. Deschler DG, Walsh KA, Friedman S, Hayden RE. Quality of life assessment in patients undergoing head and neck surgery as evaluated by lay caregivers. Laryngoscope. 1999;109(1):42–6. https://doi.org/10.1097/00005537-199901000-00009.
3. Avenanti A, Minio-Paluello I, Sforza A, Aglioti SM. Freezing or escaping? Opposite modulations of empathic reactivity to the pain of others. Cortex. 2009;45(9):1072–7. https://doi.org/10.1016/j.cortex.2008.10.004. Epub 2008 Oct 30.
4. Redelmeier DA, Dickinson VM. Judging whether a patient is actually improving: more pitfalls from the science of human perception. J Gen Intern Med. 2012;27(9):1195–9. https://doi.org/10.1007/s11606-012-2097-2. Epub 2012 May 17.
5. Bellieni CV, Cordelli DM, Raffaelli M, Ricci B, Morgese G, Buonocore G. Analgesic effect of watching TV during venipuncture. Arch Dis Child. 2006;91(12):1015–7. https://doi.org/10.1136/adc.2006.097246. Epub 2006 Aug 18.
6. Funderburk C. Best interest of the child should not be an ambiguous term. Child Legal RGT J. 2013;13:229–66.
7. Weaver MS, Lantos J, Hauschild K, Hammel J, Birge N, Janvier A. Communicating with parents of children with trisomy 13 or 18 who seek cardiac interventions. Cardiol Young. 2021;31(3):471–5. https://doi.org/10.1017/S1047951120004023. Epub 2020 Nov 19.

8. Yabrodi M, Mastropietro CW. Hypoplastic left heart syndrome: from comfort care to long-term survival. Pediatr Res. 2017;81(1–2):142–9. https://doi.org/10.1038/pr.2016.194. Epub 2016 Oct 4.
9. Kim GM, Lim JY, Kim EJ, Park SM. Resilience of patients with chronic diseases: a systematic review. Health Soc Care Community. 2019;27(4):797–807. https://doi.org/10.1111/hsc.12620. Epub 2018 Jul 20.
10. Silván-Ferrero P, Recio P, Molero F, Nouvilas-Pallejà E. Psychological quality of life in people with physical disability: the effect of internalized stigma, collective action and resilience. Int J Environ Res Public Health. 2020;17(5):1802. https://doi.org/10.3390/ijerph17051802.
11. Scheffers F, van Vugt E, Moonen X. Resilience in the face of adversity in adults with an intellectual disability: A literature review. J Appl Res Intellect Disabil. 2020;33(5):828–38.
12. Gillon R. Why Charlie Gard's parents should have been the decision-makers about their son's best interests. J Med Ethics. 2018;44(7):462–5. https://doi.org/10.1136/medethics-2017-104723. Epub 2018 May 3.
13. Janvier A, Farlow B, Barrington KJ, Bourque CJ, Brazg T, Wilfond B. Building trust and improving communication with parents of children with trisomy 13 and 18: a mixed-methods study. Palliat Med. 2020;34(3):262–71. https://doi.org/10.1177/0269216319860662. Epub 2019 Jul 8.
14. Myrhaug HT, Brurberg KG, Hov L, Markestad T. Survival and impairment of extremely premature infants: a meta-analysis. Pediatrics. 2019;143(2):e20180933. https://doi.org/10.1542/peds.2018-0933.
15. Janvier A, Barrington KJ, Aziz K, Bancalari E, Batton D, Bellieni C, Bensouda B, Blanco C, Cheung PY, Cohn F, Daboval T, Davis P, Dempsey E, Dupont-Thibodeau A, Ferretti E, Farlow B, Fontana M, Fortin-Pellerin E, Goldberg A, Hansen TW, Haward M, Kovacs L, Lapointe A, Lantos J, Morley C, Moussa A, Musante G, Nadeau S, O'Donnell CP, Orfali K, Payot A, Ryan CA, Sant'anna G, Saugstad OD, Sayeed S, Stokes TA, Verhagen E. CPS position statement for prenatal counselling before a premature birth: simple rules for complicated decisions. Paediatr Child Health. 2014;19(1):22–4.

Overcoming the Fear of Death

22.1 The Image of Death

"The idea of death, the fear of it, haunts the human animal like nothing else," wrote Earnest Becker in his book *The Denial of Death*. Death fear appears to be at the heart of several mental health disorders, including anxiety, panic disorder, and depressive disorders. We are really afraid to talk about it. A 2014 ComRes (a leading research consultancy) poll found that 8 out of 10 Britons feel uncomfortable talking about death and only a third had written a will before dying [1].

Nonetheless, the scenario is surprising when we examine it from the sick people's point of view. A recent study spread light on this theme. The researchers analyzed the writing of regular bloggers with terminal cancer or amyotrophic lateral sclerosis, who died over the course of the study; they compared them to blog posts written by a group of participants who were told to imagine of having been diagnosed with terminal cancer and of having only a few months to live. They looked for general feelings of positivity and negativity in their posts. Blog posts from terminally ill patients were found to contain considerably more positive and less negative words than they imagined, and their use of positive language increased as they neared death [2].

It is therefore necessary to review our way of thinking death. Because it is a feeling full of paradoxes. We are scared of death, but we know that it is a natural part of our existence. We are afraid of death, but when it is present, most people can face it and bear its consequences with courage.

This is very important for people in intensive care and for those entering the path of palliative care. In many cases, patients amaze us with their acceptance of disability or of a terminal prognosis. John Wyatt said, "Clinicians have a marked tendency to overestimate the impact of functional impairments and restrictions on personal well-being and life satisfaction in disabled adolescents and adults. In reality, there is no simple relationship between neurological impairment and either 'unbearable suffering' or 'poor quality of life'" [3].

So, we need to get rid of this prejudice and create an environment in which death is no longer a taboo but becomes a normal step in life. It is hard to think about it because something irrational and scary exists around the idea of death, but that's the way it is: life is made for death, and death can be accepted even when it destroys a wonderful project.

Nonetheless, death remains a mystery. And it also remains a trauma: despite any rationalization we may do, it bewilders, it overcomes and overwhelms us. The balance between people's resilience and the burden they bear for death is to be supported: the burden should not be underweighted and the resilience should be actively helped.

22.2　Rituals

End-of-life rituals should be allowed, according to the child's ethnicity, religion, or sentiment. The rituals of death are the foundations of a free and serene farewell process [4, 5]. Parents whose children die in the PICU require and appreciate assistance in obtaining a suitably "sacred" death that is peaceful and dignified. Parents require sufficient time and privacy with their child, and calm, sensitive care that honors their personality [6]. People particularly requested in these moments are holistic-health and music-therapy providers, religious or spiritual caregivers, and further family members [7]. An appropriate environment is imperative. Loud noises, laughter or insensitive comments near the baby's room are vividly remembered and regretted by the parents. Maintaining parental identity during this process is achieved through closeness to their children, respect by the staff for parents' decision-making process, their involvement in children's care, and the use of cultural and religious symbols [8]. At the time of death, the opportunity to say goodbye is essential, and its lack is a source of anguish and deep regret for the parents, often maintained for years. For the families, it is important that a staff member assist them with paperwork, contacting the funeral home, and guiding them through the next steps [9].

After death, help to be provided to the parents does not end. Inpatient memorial services are sometimes organized; they are reported to be attended by up to 60% of bereaved parents, though it is emotionally difficult for them to visit the hospital [10]. Efforts to support families and commemorate deceased children are positively valued by bereaved parents. Absences of staff members at commemorative events and lack of supportive acts are noted and deplored by families [11]. Staff members and program administrators should try to organize workloads to ensure meaningful contact between staff members and parents during the bereavement. Rituals after death can help coping with grief, provide an arena where death is recognized and accepted, create a safe place for bereaved people to express emotion, maintain a connection with other families and friends and with the deceased, and help mourning parents continue its elaboration [12]. Ritual practices after the death of a loved one include handling the remains of the deceased, organizing funeral wakes, funerals, burials, and gathering celebrations which may differ across cultures, religions, and ethnicity, socioeconomic group, and age of the deceased [13]. Knowledge of these ritual practices is important for community health nurses in providing sensitive and appropriate support to remaining family and friends.

Ritual practices for vigils, funerals, burials or cremations for an infant or child differ from those practiced for adults: services are often shorter, there are fewer prayers, cremation can be used more frequently, there are often fewer family and friends attending, and there are fewer family reunions after burials [14]. When caring for parents who have lost a baby or child, evaluate the individual needs and cultural habits of the parents as these can differ from individual to individual and from generation to generation within the same culture.

22.3 Perinatal Mourning

The concept of perinatal hospice involves that of a planned birth with the prospect of an early death; however, it can happen that the fetus dies shortly before delivery and is stillborn or dies during delivery. All this is in the scenario of perinatal bereavement. This type of bereavement must be considered and taken care of by the nursing and medical staff.

Perinatal bereavement [15] is the bereavement experienced when a child is lost during pregnancy, childbirth, or after childbirth: it is an experience of many women, which finds little space in several cultures. It is an event that deeply affects parents and can have very serious consequences on personal, couple, and family health.

Of course, in the case of stillbirth, the family will not enter into the intensive care pathway. Nevertheless, their grief should be considered; the staff of neonatal palliative care, including psychologists, and other caregivers, is particularly indicated for help them. A recent study performed in Denmark on parents of stillborn babies, reports that "Danish parents engage to a very high degree in contact with their dead baby. The analysis points out that 'Time' and 'Others' are needed to create a socially comprehensible status for parents and child when birth brings death. In liminal space during the transition, healthcare professionals act as ritual experts, supporting parents and their relatives to ascribe social status to the dead body of the child through ritualised acts. Instead of only thinking of this period as 'memory-making', we suggest regarding it as a time of ontological clarification as well" [16]. In Denmark also specialized units for perinatally bereaved parents exist in several hospitals [17]. Recent studies on the Italian perinatal palliative care situation showed performing results [18] as well as in the United States [19]. A recent editorial of Frontiers in Pediatrics so reports: "The interdisciplinary approach that PnPC [Perinatal Palliative care] brings is one of collaboration across professional disciplines, including high-risk obstetricians, neonatologists, and other specialists, in accordance with each specific diagnosis. Services to help provide comfort to the baby (lactation consultant, feeding therapists, speech pathologist, OT/PT) and emotional, psychological, and spiritual support to families (Social Work, Psychology,

Child Life, and Chaplaincy or engaging the family's faith community) are summoned to help. Yet, while there are over 300 programs of PnPC reported internationally, there is no current standard of PnPC team composition or service provision for the fragile population it addresses" [20].

Perinatal bereavement has the typical characteristics of all bereavements, and it needs help and time to be processed. After perinatal loss, bereaved couples experience distress, due to various forms of anxiety and sorrow. The minimization performed by the common Western mindset, often interferes with them grieving processes [21]. When a perinatal death happens, parents are invited by their friends and relatives to "go on," to "distract themselves," "to think in having another baby *in substitution,*" as if this sorrow were not a full sorrow. This superficiality can overshadow their mourning and their strategies to elaborate it, often labeled as "strange," "excessive," "extravagant," and "inappropriate." Although the parents have not built a full relationship with their baby, their pain does not differ significantly in intensity from other loss scenarios [22]. This amplifies the sense of isolation and loneliness of those overwhelmed by perinatal bereavement. Dealing with perinatal bereavement is not easy at all, especially for those cultures that accept evident and extroverted behaviors for bereavement and should restrain because they live in a different culture, or for the minimization that is supposed because of the age of the deceased. Mourning has a profoundly subjective dimension: parents mourn their lost loved one, their broken relationship, their projects that will not come true. Sometimes they cry for the apparent incomprehensibility of their tears, for the astonished faces of the others, for the fact that they do not understand why they are "so fond" of their children, for their sense of loneliness [23]. These expressions of suffering should not be censored just because the time spent with the baby has been so short. Bereavement should find its way and elaboration.

22.4 Assistance to the Sacredness of Life

Assistance at the level of sacredness of human life, sometimes called religious assistance, is quite distinct from psychological assistance. In fact, the latter is the support to a need that has been created as a consequence of the disease, while the former is a dimension of the human person, not limited to be described in material terms. Assistance to the sacredness of human life has two characteristics: it can be offered to anyone, considering that somebody had not or did not perceive this necessity; and it must concern the specific religious feelings of the patient. In other words, it must be free and personal, in the forms that the subject accepts and approves. This does not mean that it is an accessory, an appendix to the bereavement process. On the contrary, it should be facilitated and shared as an integrant part of the patient's and their parents' life and of the dying process.

References

1. Brown J. We fear death but what if dying isn't as bad as we think? The Guardian. 25 Jul 2017.
2. Goranson A, Ritter RS, Waytz A, Norton MI, Gray K. Dying is unexpectedly positive. Psychol Sci. 2017;28(7):988–99. https://doi.org/10.1177/0956797617701186. Epub 2017 Jun 1.
3. Wyatt J. End-of-life decisions, quality of life and the newborn. Acta Paediatr. 2007;96(6):790–1.
4. Kobler K, Limbo R, Kavanaugh K. Meaningful moments. MCN Am J Matern Child Nurs. 2007;32(5):288–95.
5. Rosenbaum JL, Smith JR, Zollfrank R. Neonatal end-of-life spiritual support care. J Perinat Neonatal Nurs. 2011;25(1):61–9. quiz 70-1. https://doi.org/10.1097/JPN.0b013e318209e1d2.
6. Davies R. Mothers' stories of loss: their need to be with their dying child and their child's body after death. J Child Health Care. 2005;9:288–300.
7. Brooten D, Youngblut JM, Seagrave L, Caicedo C, Hawthorne D, Hidalgo I, Roche R. Parent's perceptions of health care providers actions around child ICU death: what helped, what did not. Am J Hosp Palliat Care. 2013;30(1):40–9.
8. Macnab AJ, Northway T, Ryall K, et al. Death and bereavement in a paediatric intensive care unit: parental perceptions of staff support. Paediatr Child Health. 2003;8:357–62.
9. Meert KL, Briller SH, Schim SM, et al. Examining the needs of bereaved parents in the pediatric intensive care unit: a qualitative study. Death Stud. 2009;33:712–40.
10. Macdonald ME, Liben S, Carnevale FA, Rennick JE, Wolf SL, Meloche D, Cohen SR. Parental perspectives on hospital staff members' acts of kindness and commemoration after a child's death. Pediatrics. 2005;116(4):884–90. https://doi.org/10.1542/peds.2004-1980.
11. Short SR, Thienprayoon R. Pediatric palliative care in the intensive care unit and questions of quality: a review of the determinants and mechanisms of high-quality palliative care in the pediatric intensive care unit (PICU). Transl Pediatr. 2018;7(4):326–43. https://doi.org/10.21037/tp.2018.09.11.
12. Gudmundsdottir M, Chesla CA. Building a new world: habits and practices of healing following the death of a child. J Fam Nurs. 2006;12(2):143–64. https://doi.org/10.1177/1074840706287275.
13. Reeves NC. Death acceptance through ritual. Death Stud. 2011;35(5):408–19. https://doi.org/10.1080/07481187.2011.552056.
14. Cacciatore J, Ong R. Through the touch of god: child death and spiritual sustenance in a Hutterian colony. Omega (Westport). 2011–2012;64(3):185–202. https://doi.org/10.2190/om.64.3.a.
15. Fenstermacher K, Hupcey JE. Perinatal bereavement: a principle-based concept analysis. J Adv Nurs. 2013;69(11):2389–400. https://doi.org/10.1111/jan.12119. Epub 2013 Mar 4.
16. Jørgensen ML, Prinds C, Mørk S, Hvidtjørn D. Stillbirth - transitions and rituals when birth brings death: data from a Danish national cohort seen through an anthropological lens. Scand J Caring Sci. 2022;36(1):100–8. https://doi.org/10.1111/scs.12967.
17. Hvidtjørn D, Mørk S, Eklund M, Maimburg RD, Henriksen TB. Women's length of stay in a Danish specialized unit for perinatally bereaved parents. J Obstet Gynecol Neonatal Nurs. 2021;50(6):714–23. https://doi.org/10.1016/j.jogn.2021.06.009.
18. Locatelli C, Corvaglia L, Simonazzi G, Bisulli M, Paolini L, Faldella G. "Percorso Giacomo": an Italian innovative service of perinatal palliative care. Front Pediatr. 2020;8:589559. https://doi.org/10.3389/fped.2020.589559.
19. Wool C, Parravicini E. The neonatal comfort care program: origin and growth over 10 years. Front Pediatr. 2020;8:588432. https://doi.org/10.3389/fped.2020.588432.
20. Carter BS, Parravicini E, Benini F, Lago P. Editorial: perinatal palliative care comes of age. Front Pediatr. 2021;9:709383. https://doi.org/10.3389/fped.2021.709383.

21. Lang A, Fleiszer AR, Duhamel F, Sword W, Gilbert KR, Corsini-Munt S. Perinatal loss and parental grief: the challenge of ambiguity and disenfranchised grief. Omega (Westport). 2011;63(2):183–96.
22. Kersting A, Wagner B. Complicated grief after perinatal loss. Dialogues Clin Neurosci. 2012;14(2):187–94. https://doi.org/10.31887/DCNS.2012.14.2/akersting.
23. Moore T, Parrish H, Black BP. Interconception care for couples after perinatal loss: a comprehensive review of the literature. J Perinat Neonatal Nurs. 2011;25(1):44–51. https://doi.org/10.1097/JPN.0b013e3182071a08.

Part VII
Types of Pediatric Palliative Care

Pediatric palliative care has several ways for being applied. Here, we describe them carefully, inviting caregivers to choose the best option for each case. We have the possibility of choosing home care, community-based home care, hospice-care, and palliative care within the intensive care unit setting. Unfortunately, not all forms here described are available worldwide. All these features testify the high level of specialistic development this branch of medicine has attained.

Territorial Differentiation and Home Care

23.1 The Mission of Pediatric Palliative Care

Pediatric palliative care aims to take care of families' physical, psychosocial, and spiritual problems from a family-centered perspective, providing continuity of care that connects different events and places of care. For nearly 15 years, the American Academy of Pediatrics has argued that all children with life-threatening illnesses should receive access to palliative care in an integrated system, offering palliative care from diagnosis and throughout the course of the disease, regardless of whether the outcome is recovery or death [1]. In 2016, the World Health Organization recommended broadening the scope of palliative care beyond end-of-life cases, to children living with complex chronic conditions, those at high risk of mortality, significant morbidity, cases complicated by conflict on the goals of care, difficult symptom control, anticipated and prolonged hospitalization, frequent re-admission, and staff moral distress [2]. The core principles of pediatric palliative care, namely symptom relief, quality of life, communication, relationship building, and targeted decision-making, focus on interdisciplinary collaboration to address these issues from multiple perspectives [3]. In an optimal family-centered model, pediatric palliative care begins at the time of diagnosis of a life-threatening condition and is introduced as another supporting pillar within the standard of care paradigm [4]. Once integrated into the child's management plan, pediatric palliative care extends throughout the trajectory of the disease, slipping between inpatient and outpatient facilities, to promote the continuity of care [5].

The basic principles of palliative care, such as attention to the burden of symptoms and considerations on the quality of life, fall within the competence of intensive care practitioners and constitute "primary palliative care." However, in the case of complex decision-making, complicated bereavement, care transitions, and a high symptom burden, intensivists may seek the experience of the palliativist. The palliative care service serves ICU families needing additional psychosocial support, as well as those needing home assistance and those requiring referral to a hospice [2].

23.2 Types of Approach

From an organizational point of view, there are theoretically three possible solutions for children with very serious or terminal diseases. They are the hospital set, mainly in the case of intensive care or acute diseases, pediatric/neonatal hospices, and home assistance. None of these solutions are ideal; basically, they all have their pros and cons.

The hospital service plays an essential role in identifying children and families in need, which includes integrating the palliative approach within the hospital, liaising effectively with community-based services, and providing impeccable assessment and treatment of pain and other problems to the betterment of the mind, body, and spirit of children and their families [6]. Palliative care provided in hospitals is practiced by a team of expert intensivists, with formal training in pediatric palliative care; they work within an interdisciplinary team model to maximize patients' quality of life, while addressing physical, psychosocial needs, and spirituality of patients and families (Fig. 23.1) [7].

The hospice has the advantage of providing the skills in the management of rare and complex cases far from the hospital set, guaranteeing sufficiently large numbers of hospitalizations to allow to provide the necessary professional skills and have sufficient economic resources; but it has the disadvantage of separating children from their environment. A particular form of pediatric hospice is the perinatal hospice, which also involves the professional figures of obstetricians, midwives, and geneticists [8].

Fig. 23.1 The dynamics of pediatric palliative care. The four approaches here illustrated, dynamically integrate each other in a global pediatric palliative care (PPC)

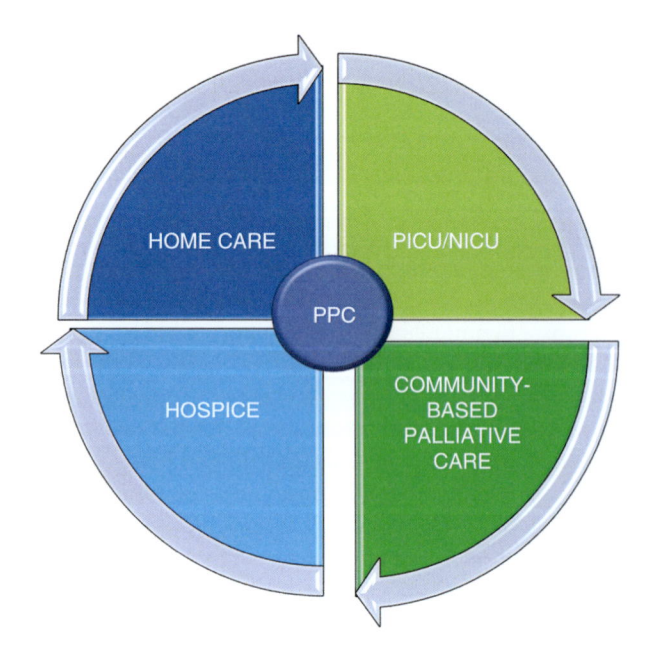

Alongside these advantages, there is the discomfort of the family, which would like to return to live the child's illness at home. Staying at home can certainly satisfy a patient's request, but it has its drawbacks: operators specialized in the child's disease can only reach a limited part of the territory. If the children to be cared for are numerous and distant from each other, it is difficult—in organizational and economic terms—to implement home care outside the big cities, where the population density is higher. Keeping patients at home in an integrated home care system returns children to their families and social settings, receiving multidisciplinary services at home, but again the primary burden of patient management and support often falls primarily on the family [9].

Community-based pediatric palliative care can be managed through home care or hospice agencies or other specialist physicians present and organized in the community, with support provided in person, by phone or by email [10, 11].

Thus, all the assistance possibilities just described have strengths and weaknesses. The pediatric palliative care models currently adopted use a combination of the three types described above, considering them almost as organizational modules within a single support network, in which different health institutions and families are involved at different times during the illness of the patient, giving priority to one or the other type of solution according to the patient's condition and specific situations.

23.3　Home Care

Spending the latter part of life at home seems to be the best option for children; this is not so obvious. A systematic review highlighted the complexity of home palliative care experiences of families [12]: whether they prefer hospitals or their own home as their last place of care depends on the facilities offered, the distance of the service from home, the availability of home care, and the type of disease [12]. Families receiving pediatric palliative care need organized and individualized support from a specialized pediatric palliative care team. They need respite, to manage a challenging home care situation, and support for their siblings. However, a recent review that analyzed the demands of children and families when receiving palliative care at home showed that most families preferred to stay at home as it made it easier to maintain a normal family life, was less stressful for the sick child and meant that the siblings could still attend school and be with friends. Many children report wanting to stay at home [13], so that schoolmates can drop by for a visit on their way home from school and grandparents could come for dinner, give their support, and spend time with their grandchildren. Commuting to the hospital and vice versa takes time and energy [13]: if health workers could come to the children's homes, the sick child could spend his or her precious time and energy on more interesting activities, rather than on travels, sometimes made only for minor procedures.

It seems paradoxical that, while the ability to have more rest is a strong point of home care [14], the difficult access to care resources makes respite nearly impossible. Therefore, the support of competent home palliative care teams, which also takes into account the rhythms and needs of family dynamics, is an important factor in promoting well-being and increasing the quality of life of families at home [15], and consequently their respite. Several studies report difficulties and benefits of home palliative care in neonatal age. Parents report feeling alone in their grief and struggling to cope with their partners' different style of grief; their primary concerns after hospital discharge include transporting their child/baby home, feeding them, changing cranial device dressings, managing pain and seizures, addressing uncertainty, and facilitating a good death [16]. Shandeigh Berry, in a study on anencephalic babies cared at home, reported that all parents "received hospice services from healthcare professionals without perinatal bereavement training or experience. Only one woman received follow-up care after the death of her son" [16].

Thus, a possible option is an integration of home assistance with the territorial healthcare assistance. Unfortunately, this is not always possible: pediatric palliative care is still underdeveloped and the same is true for community-integrated palliative care. Few countries have a satisfying palliative care organization. Poor development of community-integrated palliative care health services and bureaucratizing processes are obstacles for families, with the result that the child encounters so many obstacles that they end up dying in hospital rather than at home [17]. Moreover, the financial and logistic support families need when assisting a complex child at home is great but often absent. Unfortunately, studies aimed at assessing the costs undergone by families of children with life-limiting diseases who treat their child at home are small and inconsistent [18].

23.4 Community-Based Pediatric Palliative Care

Community-based pediatric palliative care is a branch of pediatric palliative care that connects hospice, home, and hospital facilities; thus, community-based pediatric palliative care programs play a vital role in coordinating and delivering complex care for children with life-threatening conditions and their families [10]. There is a difference between community palliative care and "home care" or "home palliative care"; palliative care outside a protected hospital structure should not become a mere family affair: as it affects the health of patients, they require a community response. Health must never be a private phenomenon, with social disinterest and sometimes with the isolation of the patient.

Almost 20 years ago, the Institute of Medicine published a report titled "Improving Palliative and End of Life Care for Children," calling for improvements in community pediatric palliative care through better collaboration between individual healthcare professionals, pediatric hospitals, home care services, and hospices [19]. In September 2014, the Institute of Medicine published another comprehensive analysis of the current state of end-of-life care in America, in which it again advocated better access to home care as a means of achieving a higher quality of life. including improved listening and communication, emotional and spiritual support, well-being and dignity, death assistance, and a lighter symptom load [10, 20]. Supported by these consensus statements, many have endorsed the inclusion of

23.4 Community-Based Pediatric Palliative Care

pediatric home palliative care services as a key component of an effective holistic care model [21]. Collaboration and trust between healthcare professionals and parents, and within healthcare teams, are required for effective palliative home management of pediatric pain; community healthcare professionals require specialized education to effectively manage pediatric pain at home, end of life, and to prevent emergency hospital admissions, as was positively experienced during the recent COVID19 pandemic [22].

Pediatric Cancer Centers provide and set basic therapy in adolescents and children, who often return home to continue therapy and receive palliative care: community-based pediatric palliative care facilitates this transition and improves the overall home experience. Unfortunately, the community-based pediatric home palliative care network is not yet widespread [23]. Despite advances, early integration of pediatric palliative care into the hospital, not to mention community-based pediatric palliative care, appears to be practiced inconsistently across most of the world cure centers as a standard of care in the management of children with cancer [10, 24]. However, integrating community-based pediatric palliative care principles and services for pediatric cancer patients is not just a compassionate practice; it is an evidence-based imperative component of care [10]. In particular, the involvement of community-based pediatric palliative care in the care of children with cancer improves symptom management [25], quality of life [26], and other valuable outcomes for children and their families are suggested. Although current models of pediatric palliative care take place primarily in the hospital setting, community-based pediatric palliative care programs are increasingly in demand [10]. Parents of children with life-threatening conditions who used community pediatric palliative care services prior to their child's death, described their death as "very peaceful," reporting that the involvement of community pediatric palliative care led to very significant improvements in the symptoms and quality of life of the child, improvement of communication aspects, and reduction of administrative barriers [27]. Parents also reported very significant improvements in their quality of life, with fewer reports of psychological distress [27]. Healthcare professionals themselves have also reported significant improvements in all fields of care, particularly in the areas of cooperation, communication, and family support [27].

In addition to the aforementioned proven benefits gained from involvement before the death, community-based pediatric palliative care also significantly improves the death experience for children and families. Parents of children with life-threatening conditions are increasingly reporting a preference for their child's death to occur at home [28], and community-based pediatric palliative care services have been shown to increase the rate of children dying at home according to the wishes of the family [29, 30]. In this way, community-based pediatric palliative care programs benefit not only the child and family wishing to stay at home, but also potentially the affiliated hospital, which can be fiscally incentivized to reduce frequent or long hospitalizations. Data also suggests that terminally ill children spend most of their last 6 months of life at home [31]. In these cases, community-based pediatric palliative care can give a substantial contribution to the care and well-being of these children and their families.

The economic benefit of community pediatric palliative care should not be underestimated when assessing its implementation. This type of care can lead to a reduction in the length of hospital stay and emergency care, and therefore to a reduction in overall hospital costs. [32]. Therefore, it is reasonable to believe that providing high-quality home-based pediatric palliative care has the potential to reduce healthcare costs by minimizing re-hospitalization in selected children with life-threatening conditions. As terminal care models remain key cost-drivers in the current healthcare model, the subsidy to community-based pediatric palliative care resources could produce significant tax savings in this context [33].

References

1. American Academy of Pediatrics. Committee on Bioethics and Committee on Hospital Care. Palliative care for children. Pediatrics. 2000;106(2 pt 1):351–7.
2. World Health Organization. Integrating palliative care and symptom relief into paediatrics: a WHO guide for health care planners, implementers and managers. Geneva: World Health Organization; 2018. Accessed on May 5th 2022. https://apps.who.int/iris/handle/10665/274561
3. Levine D, Lam CG, Cunningham MJ, et al. Best practices for pediatric palliative cancer care: a primer for clinical providers. J Support Oncol. 2013;11:114–125.
4. Friebert S, Osenga K. Pediatric palliative care referral criteria. New York: Center to Advance Palliative Care; 2009. Accessed 1 Sept 2014.
5. Ullrich CK, Wolfe J. Caring for children living with life-threatening illness: a growing relationship between pediatric hospital medicine and pediatric palliative care. Pediatr Clin N Am. 2014;61:xxi–xxiii.
6. Drake R. Palliative care for children in hospital: essential roles. Children (Basel). 2018;5(2):26. https://doi.org/10.3390/children5020026.
7. Snaman J, McCarthy S, Wiener L, Wolfe J. Pediatric palliative care in oncology. J Clin Oncol. 2020;38(9):954–62. https://doi.org/10.1200/JCO.18.02331. Epub 2020 Feb 5.
8. Mixer SJ, Lindley L, Wallace H, Fornehed ML, Wool C. The relationship between the nursing environment and delivering culturally sensitive perinatal hospice care. Int J Palliat Nurs. 2015;21(9):423–9. https://doi.org/10.12968/ijpn.2015.21.9.423.
9. Benini F, Spizzichino M, Trapanotto M, et al. Pediatric palliative care. Ital J Pediatr. 2008;34:4.
10. Kaye EC, Rubenstein J, Levine D, Baker JN, Dabbs D, Friebert SE. Pediatric palliative care in the community. CA Cancer J Clin. 2015;65(4):316–33.
11. Lindley LC, Keim-Malpass J, Svynarenko R, Cozad MJ, Mack JW, Hinds PS. Pediatric concurrent hospice care: a scoping review and directions for future nursing research. J Hosp Palliat Nurs. 2020;22(3):238–45. https://doi.org/10.1097/NJH.0000000000000648.
12. Bluebond-Langner M, Beecham E, Candy B, Langner R, Jones L. Preferred place of death for children and young people with life-limiting and life-threatening conditions: a systematic review of the literature and recommendations for future inquiry and policy. Palliat Med. 2013;27(8):705.
13. Castor C, Landgren K, Hansson H, Kristensson HI. A possibility for strengthening family life and health: family members' lived experience when a sick child receives home care in Sweden. Health Soc Care Community. 2018;26(2):224–31.
14. Ling J. Respite support for children with a life-limiting condition and their parents: a literature review. Int J Palliat Nurs. 2012;18(3):129–34. https://doi.org/10.12968/ijpn.2012.18.3.129. PMID: 22584313.
15. Winger A, Kvarme LG, Løyland B, Kristiansen C, Helseth S, Ravn IH. Family experiences with palliative care for children at home: a systematic literature review. BMC Palliat Care. 2020;19(1):165. https://doi.org/10.1186/s12904-020-00672-4.

References

16. Berry SN. Providing palliative care to neonates with anencephaly in the home setting. J Hosp Palliat Nurs. 2021;23(4):367–74. https://doi.org/10.1097/NJH.0000000000000770.
17. Mariyana R, Allenidekania A, Nurhaeni N. Parents' voice in managing the pain of children with cancer during palliative care. Indian J Palliat Care. 2018;24(2):156–61. https://doi.org/10.4103/IJPC.IJPC_198_17.
18. Mitterer S, Zimmermann K, Bergsträsser E, Simon M, Gerber AK, Fink G. Measuring financial burden in families of children living with life-limiting conditions: a scoping review of cost indicators and outcome measures. Value Health. 2021;24(9):1377–89. https://doi.org/10.1016/j.jval.2021.03.015. Epub 2021 Aug 7.
19. Institute of Medicine of the National Academies. In: Field MJ, Behrman RE, editors. When children die: improving palliative and end-of-life care for children and their families. Washington, DC: The National Academies Press; 2003.
20. Institute of Medicine (US) Committee on Palliative and End-of-Life Care for Children and Their Families; Field MJ, Behrman RE, editors. When Children Die: Improving Palliative and End-of-Life Care for Children and Their Families. Washington (DC): National Academies Press (US); 2003. APPENDIX E, BEREAVEMENT EXPERIENCES AFTER THE DEATH OF A CHILD. Available at: https://www.ncbi.nlm.nih.gov/books/NBK220798/.
21. Boyden JY, Curley MAQ, Deatrick JA, Ersek M. Factors associated with the use of U.S. community-based palliative care for children with life-limiting or life-threatening illnesses and their families: an integrative review. J Pain Symptom Manag. 2018;55(1):117–31. https://doi.org/10.1016/j.jpainsymman.2017.04.017. Epub 2017 Aug 12.
22. Greenfield DK, Carter B, Harrop DE, Jassal DS, Bayliss MJ, Renton DK, Holley DS, Howard DRF, Johnson MM, Liossi C. Healthcare professionals' experiences of the barriers and facilitators to pediatric pain management in the community at end-of-life: a qualitative interview study. J Pain Symptom Manage. 2022;63(1):98–105. https://doi.org/10.1016/j.jpainsymman.2021.06.026.
23. Abu Sharour LM, Al-Noumani H, Al SS, Al HI, Al HM, Al-Yazidi B. Community-based palliative care in the Arab region: current status and future directions. In: Silbermann M, editor. Palliative care for chronic cancer patients in the community. Cham: Springer; 2021.
24. Johnston DL, Vadeboncoeur C. Palliative care consultation in pediatric oncology. Support Care Cancer. 2012;20:799–803.
25. Schmidt P, Otto M, Hechler T, Metzing S, Wolfe J, Zernikow B. Did increased availability of pediatric palliative care lead to improved palliative care outcomes in children with cancer? J Palliat Med. 2013;16:1034–39.
26. Groh G, Borasio GD, Nickolay C, Bender HU, von Lüttichau I, Führer M. Specialized pediatric palliative home care: a prospective evaluation. J Palliat Med. 2013;16(12):1588–94. https://doi.org/10.1089/jpm.2013.0129. Epub 2013 Oct 29.
27. Vollenbroich R, Duroux A, Grasser M, Brandstätter M, Borasio GD, Führer M. Effectiveness of a pediatric palliative home care team as experienced by parents and health care professionals. J Palliat Med. 2012;15(3):294–300. https://doi.org/10.1089/jpm.2011.0196. Epub 2012 Jan 4.
28. Ullrich CK, Dussel V, Hilden JM, Sheaffer JW, Lehmann L, Wolfe J. End-of-life experience of children undergoing stem cell transplantation for malignancy: parent and provider perspectives and patterns of care. Blood. 2010;115(19):3879–85. https://doi.org/10.1182/blood-2009-10-250225. Epub 2010 Mar 12.
29. Feudtner C, DiGiuseppe DL, Neff JM. Hospital care for children and young adults in the last year of life: a population-based study. BMC Med. 2003;1:3. https://doi.org/10.1186/1741-7015-1-3.
30. Feudtner C, Feinstein JA, Satchell M, Zhao H, Kang TI. Shifting place of death among children with complex chronic conditions in the United States, 1989-2003. JAMA. 2007;297(24):2725–32. https://doi.org/10.1001/jama.297.24.2725.
31. Niswander LM, Cromwell P, Chirico J, Gupton A, Korones DN. End-of-life care for children enrolled in a community-based pediatric palliative care program. J Palliat Med. 2014;17(5):589–91.

32. Postier A, Chrastek J, Nugent S, Osenga K, Friedrichsdorf SJ. Exposure to home-based pediatric palliative and hospice care and its impact on hospital and emergency care charges at a single institution. J Palliat Med. 2014;17(2):183–8. https://doi.org/10.1089/jpm.2013.0287. Epub 2013 Dec 31.
33. Chirico J, Donnelly JP, Gupton A, Cromwell P, Miller M, Dawson C, Korones DN. Costs of care and location of death in community-based pediatric palliative care. J Palliat Med. 2019;22(5):517–21. https://doi.org/10.1089/jpm.2018.0276. Epub 2019 Feb 7.

The Pediatric Hospices

24.1 The Pediatric Hospice

The pediatric hospice is an important ring in the pediatric palliative care chain: it is a highly complex facility, designed for the child; often open-space, adapted to specific age groups, giving children the opportunity to socialize and providing the skills and the social interactions that can help the patient lead a "normal life." It can be the connecting bridge between hospital and home, or it can temporarily give the family the opportunity to take a break from the burden of care, when the family needs help for some reason, or when the clinical management of the patient becomes too complex. It is not a place where patients go just before they die; it is a reference point that continuously interacts in the healthcare network at a clinical, educational, and research level. The environment of a hospice can be defined as "prosthetic" for the patient [1] because it provides an extension of those skills have been weakened in the baby/child: frequenting school, playing, walking in some cases. Although caring for a sick or dying child may focus on palliation, active treatment is also part of palliative care in the hospice, and both aspects play an important role during a child's illness.

Adult hospice is often devoted to the care of the terminally ill, and in the United States a prognosis of 6 months or less is required for insurance approval of the hospice benefit; however, children use hospices longer than adults [2]. Prognosis-based hospices may not be appropriate for children, as children may receive hospice services and curative or life-prolonging therapies at the same time [3]. US data indicate that 78% of adult hospices provide pediatric care, with an average of less than 20 children [4]; the pediatric hospice has its own peculiarities because it is usually concerned with rare diseases, or with dubious diagnosis or prognosis [5], so that their increment is therefore auspicable.

Pediatric hospices are not still widespread across the world, also because of the scarce diffusion of pediatric palliative care itself. The ratio of adult palliative care specialists to pediatric palliative care specialists is about 20:1 in England [6].

© The Author(s), under exclusive license to Springer Nature Switzerland AG 2022
C. V. Bellieni, *A New Holistic-Evolutive Approach to Pediatric Palliative Care*,
https://doi.org/10.1007/978-3-030-96256-2_24

Hospices still find resistances: palliative care is still identified with end-of-life and the healthcare system comes to it when it is often too late; furthermore, children and families, if they can, choose to spend the end-of-life period at their home. Nonetheless, this does not indicate a uselessness of hospices: the possibility of choosing between home and hospice is always seen with relief and gratitude [7], and it is obvious that such an offer could not be proposed if there were no hospice beds. Furthermore, the services hospices can offer are not limited to hospital care for families who choose to spend their last days there. In hospices, families typically encounter a range of complementary therapies that hospitals are usually unable to provide.

24.2 Perinatal Hospices

The goal of perinatal palliative care is to address and support the family which has received a troubling, life-limiting, or life-threatening fetal diagnosis [8]. Perinatal hospices are a part of this road. This particular type of pediatric hospices implies taking in charge the pregnancy and the parents expecting a child who, through prenatal diagnosis, has been predicted to survive shortly after birth. It is important having an already established path of collaboration between gynecologists, obstetricians, geneticists, and neonatologists, to provide all the necessary information to the family: who make the prenatal diagnosis should not be the only consultant who takes the burden of talking about prognosis and of the treatments the child-to-be requires. The first one who makes the diagnosis cannot be always adequate for treating all types of prenatal diseases. At birth, the baby with a life-limiting pathology will be received by the neonatology staff, together with the family; after the necessary medical treatments, they will be roomed in the perinatal hospice, an environment equal to that of the pediatric hospice, especially equipped for baby care [9].

24.3 Architectural and Structural Guidelines of Pediatric Hospices

Hospices are not improvised. Their structure must be well thought out and elaborated. In fact, spaces and their components influence human activities, contributing to determining positive or negative effects on the living conditions, and the consequent level of quality of life of individuals, social groups, and communities [10]. A depressing environment gets depressed, one with architectural barriers emphasizes disability and stigmatizes it. But the environment can help; it can improve the child's mood and compliance; therefore, it has been defined as prosthetic, as if it were a prosthesis, an extension of the body and an accomplice of its needs: an essential element of well-being for patients, family members, and healthcare professionals [11].

The environment can be designed and built adequately only if there is a deep knowledge of the psychological aspects of the type its future users. The quality of the spaces is strictly connected, firstly, with the recognition of the needs to be guaranteed and, secondly, with the important role played by the habits, preferences, or limitations of the users. Only those who live the everyday life of a place can build respecting its history and its tenants; we can say that "dwelling" precedes "building"; thus, primarily those who experience the pediatric intensive care and hospices as a patient or as an operator can speak about the needs of necessary structures, and must therefore be listened to; this is not a possible option but an obligation.

In a recent study [1], the level of satisfaction of experts and users about several pediatric hospices in northern Italy was assessed. Several proposals have emerged that we report here, as fundamental or at least highly desirable points for a hospice, that coincide with hints appeared in literature.

Complementary Therapies: therapies offered in pediatric hospices, ranging from music and art therapy to pets, with the exception of hydrotherapy, received staff satisfaction scores ranging from 7 to 9/10.

Room spaces: according to this study, pediatric hospices should have less than 10 beds, characterized by good architectural, functional, and sanitary flexibility. The child's room must be above the standard requirements, and for this purpose it is necessary to design the hospital unit as mono-apartments consisting of semi-autonomous rooms of about 40 m^2 [1].

The view of the external world should be guaranteed [12].

Green areas: one of the most common proposals discussed by professionals is the integration of a green space within the building that allows for visual or active use. The presence of green spaces, such as curative gardens, plays a key role in the process of humanizing spaces in a patient-centered approach [13, 14].

Privacy: the structure must be centered on the child and their family, dedicating one or two rooms to the confidentiality and privacy of the family; the environment must give the possibility to prepare and consume meals inside, it must also have meeting spaces for relatives, as well as rooms for the necessary therapies. Everything must guarantee privacy.

Architectural barriers: a horizontal development is necessary to facilitate orientation and usability by people with disabilities or neurological diseases [1].

References

1. Gola M, Francalanza PC, Galloni G, Pagella B, Capolongo S. Architectures for paediatric palliative care: how to improve quality of life and environmental Well-being. Ann Ist Super Sanita. 2016;52(1):48–55. https://doi.org/10.4415/ANN_16_01_10.
2. Friebert S, Williams C. NHPCO's Facts and Figures. Pediatric Palliative & Hospice Care in America. 2015; Edition. Available at: https://www.nhpco.org/wp-content/uploads/2019/04/Pediatric_Facts-Figures.pdf. Accessed on May 5th 2022.
3. Rosenbaum S. The Patient Protection and Affordable Care Act: implications for public health policy and practice. Public Health Rep. 2011;126(1):130–5. https://doi.org/10.1177/003335491112600118.
4. Short SR, Thienprayoon R. Pediatric palliative care in the intensive care unit and questions of quality: a review of the determinants and mechanisms of high-quality palliative care in

the pediatric intensive care unit (PICU). Transl Pediatr. 2018;7(4):326–43. https://doi.org/10.21037/tp.2018.09.11.
5. Dingfield L, Bender L, Harris P, et al. Comparison of pediatric and adult hospice patients using electronic medical record data from nine hospices in the United States, 2008-2012. J Palliat Med. 2015;18:120–6.
6. Hain RDW. Hospices and palliative care for children: converging stories. Br Med Bull. 2019;130(1):81–8. https://doi.org/10.1093/bmb/ldz012.
7. Boyden JY, Curley MAQ, Deatrick JA, Ersek M. Factors Associated With the Use of U.S. Community-Based Palliative Care for Children With Life-Limiting or Life-Threatening Illnesses and Their Families: An Integrative Review. J Pain Symptom Manage. 2018;55(1):117–31.
8. Carter BS, Parravicini E, Benini F, Lago P. Editorial: perinatal palliative care comes of age. Front Pediatr. 2021;9:709383. https://doi.org/10.3389/fped.2021.709383.
9. Tucker MH, Ellis K, Linebarger J. Outcomes following perinatal palliative care consultation: a retrospective review. J Perinatol. 2021;41(9):2196–200. https://doi.org/10.1038/s41372-021-00966-2.
10. Evans GW, McCoy JM. When buildings don't work: the role of architecture in human health. J Environ Psychol. 1998;18(1):85–94.
11. Guaita A, Jones M. A "prosthetic" approach for individuals with dementia? JAMA. 2011;305(4):402–3. https://doi.org/10.1001/jama.2011.28.
12. van Oel CJ, Mlihi M, Freeke A. Design models for single patient rooms tested for patient preferences. HERD. 2021;14(1):31-46. doi: https://doi.org/10.1177/1937586720937995. Epub 2020 Jul 14.
13. Buffoli M, Capolongo S, Cattaneo M, Signorelli C. Project, natural lighting and comfort indoor. Ann Ig. 2007;19(5):429–41.
14. Ulrich RS. Natural versus urban scenes: some psychophysiological effects. Environ Behav. 1981;13:523–56.

Palliative Care Integrated in the Hospital Ward and the Abundance Medicine

25.1 The Limits of Intensive Set for Palliative Care

The intensive care set, which is hectic and noisy, is not the best place to get palliative care which, of course, orbits around compassion and relaxation. It's not a mission impossible to merge the two scenarios, saving the best of both, but it's not that easy. Therefore, should the child remain in pediatric intensive care, the intervention of a palliativist is desirable. The involvement of the palliativist takes place as an external consultant, or integrated into the intensive care team. The advantages exist for both models. However, in a recent study, the intensivists indicate a reluctance to "consult" the palliative care provider, fearing that parents perceive palliative care as a "renunciation" and that the palliative care team gives indications that conflict with their own [1]. The most frequently cited reasons are: (a) excessive personal confidence in personally addressing the palliative care needs of patients, (b) poor visibility of palliative care practitioners within the hospital unit intensive care, (c) an often small staff dedicated to palliative care, with the exception of the largest centers [1].

The emotional burden, the problems of ethical choices and burnout represent barriers to the provision of palliative care by the intensive care staff. Nurses and doctors in intensive care facilities already bear the burden of urgently treating the sick, alleviating their suffering with common tools, accommodating the wishes of the families and providing a modicum of peace in an intensive care environment. You can hardly ask them to do more. The high-intensity nature of the ICU and the time requirements of the intensivists represent obstacles to the practice of palliative care.

However, intensivists can do a lot in the palliative field without excessively increasing their burden of work: mitigating moral distress by allowing family support, discussing with the child and family members, clarifying the goals of treatments, coordinating communication between the medical team and the family. However, intensive care requires time and gives stress; this is one of the reasons why

© The Author(s), under exclusive license to Springer Nature Switzerland AG 2022
C. V. Bellieni, *A New Holistic-Evolutive Approach to Pediatric Palliative Care*, https://doi.org/10.1007/978-3-030-96256-2_25

pediatric intensive care workers demonstrate poor management of symptoms related to palliative care and even, understandably, cases of non-recognition of patients' delirium, dyspnea, nausea, discharge, agitation, and psychological symptoms are reported [1]. As many as 60% of parents in one study reported poor judgment by their doctors regarding the management of terminal symptoms in the ICU, including pain [2]. The climate of constant alarm of the ICU has a negative impact on the stress of parents, who, in making decisions, sometimes feel excluded and perceive the loss of their parental role, especially in the presence of language barriers. Stress is minor in parents who have been involved in babies' care and are well informed.

Intensivists could do a lot in the palliative field; nonetheless, the intensivists' knowledge of the principles of palliative care and the perception of their role in managing symptoms of stress and suffering and in decision-making—which fall within the scope of palliation—is variable and sometimes inadequate [3]. Knowledge of the legal issues of terminal pediatric care, and in particular of ethical ones, are sometimes generic among intensivists [4]. Finally, the intensive care unit alone is largely unable to prevent a serious parenting outcome: complicated bereavement, a phenomenon that occurs in up to 60% of parents with seriously ill children in the intensive care unit. Rarely post-death follow-up is offered by the critical care team for bereaved parents [1]. Also both doctors and parents confuse palliative care with end of life [5]. But this is not the case everywhere; for example, to overcome this obstacle, some ICUs have renamed their palliative care team as "Comprehensive Care," "Supportive Care," "Quality of Life," or "Advanced Care" so that palliative care is perceived as part of the "routine" of intensive care.

25.2 Pediatric Intensive Care Units: Improvements

Children with a necessity of palliative care, should find even in the pediatric intensive care unit an environment tailored on their exigencies, and those of their families. Some elements that make a hospital a "humanized" site and adapted to palliative care needs are its morphology, light, color, smell, sound, synesthesia, art, privacy, and individuality. But also the absence of noise, of excessive lights, hastiness, sleep disruption, contact with possibly toxic substances. Most of these elements are mentioned in Florence Nightingale's environmental theory, which—though ancient in time—makes it a reference for health unit building projects focused on humanization. Florence Nightingale was the pioneer of gentle and personalized care for hospitalized patients. Some of her remarks are still valid today and can make the PICU environment more palliative-care-friendly.

- First of all, the importance she gave to the hospital environment as an essential factor for care. Her idea of ideal environment followed three axes: the environment as a meeting space between individuals, as a facilitating tool of the caregivers' work, and as comfort [6]. Nightingale stressed that if one or more aspects of an environment are unbalanced, the patient uses more energy to counterbalance

the environmental stress; the nurse must intervene to identify any imbalances in the environment to harmonize the energy, putting the patient in the best situation, so that nature acts on him, favoring their recovery [7].
- Regarding noise, Nightingale indicated the need to observe silence [7]. We know that pediatric intensive care units are environments where there is too much noise, due to alarms from monitors, equipment, doorbells, telephones, televisions, and noises from communication between professionals. It is recommended that noise levels do not exceed 45 dB; and, in the pediatric intensive care units, the use of sound-absorbing walls and floors should be adopted. Furthermore, exposure to high noise levels can impact on nurses' and doctors' productivity [8]. Reducing noise levels may reduce anxiety and stress in patients and staff and can reduce sleep deprivation. Sleep deprivation is common in ICU patients and may have detrimental effects on the recovery process. Research is in progress on the use of white sound to control environment noise [9].
- It is worth remembering that in pediatric intensive care settings, in addition to the use of colors, the environment must have childish features. We have many examples, such as the "Aquarium Carioca" of the Institute of Childcare and Pediatrics of Martagão Gesteira—Instituto de Puericultura and Pediatrics Martagão Gesteira (IPPMG) and the Submarino Carioca project of the Jesus Municipal Hospital, both located in the city of Rio de Janeiro. Data from a study on school-age children reveal that they would like the PICU to be more colorful and decorated with both abstract and infantile motifs [10].
- Florence Nightingale established in her studies that the distance between the beds should not allow the stagnation of air and should favor the movement of people for the simultaneous execution of the procedures. The measurements she suggested are 4.5 m for the height of the ceiling with 3.5 m between the opposite beds [6]. Echoing these recommendations, today it is recommended that rooms are wide and airy. Beds arranged along long hallways are the least efficient configuration; square, triangular, or radial plans are often more effective. The Health Building Note [11] of the British Health Service recommends 26 m^2/bed. In the multi-bed areas, beds should be positioned to maximize patient privacy. Hand washing facilities should be available for each bed. In view of the increasing number of surgical interventions that take place at the bedside, a surgical scrub sink should be installed for every eight beds [9].
- Particular attention should be paid to the materials used for the rooms and the instruments that come into contact with the children. Too often, they are made of potentially toxic substances such as phthalates, molecules used to make plastics soft, and which are found in catheters, tracheal tubes, stethoscopes, transfusion bags, and linoleum [12] that should be replaced by phthalate-free materials.

The lack of these features makes it difficult - if not impossible - a relaxed and safe staying in hospital for children with the need of palliative care. The English Pediatric Intensive Care Society says: "Children who are critically ill or injured have specific play and psychological needs that should be addressed by specialist programs of care that are vital in meeting their overall holistic needs and their fundamental right to play" [9]. So, it is of fundamental importance to provide the basic features that we have detailed here, about the risks of physical pollution and all the possibilities of humanization of the environment.

25.3 The Neonatal Intensive Care Unit

All we have detailed for pediatric intensive care wards can be repeated for neonatal wards; obviously in this case, we will not have beds, but incubators; also here, we find recommendations for the spaces to be kept available to each baby, spaces for the mother, spaces for technical materials and for health professionals. But the importance of an environment tailored on the newborn's exigencies and on their families is crucial, maybe even more than in the case of older children, since these babies are more sensible to external stressors. The fact that they seem "protected" within incubators and isolated from the exterior world is only appearance: noises, lights, even electromagnetic fields, and the exposure to toxic substances can harass the baby even and particularly within the walls of an incubator [13, 14]: within neonatal incubators, noises can exceed 100 dB when a porthole is closed abruptly [15].

We recommend to strictly vigil the level of stress babies undergo: since they cannot claim for their health, it is our duty to stand by them and for them. Excesses in blood examinations, transfusions, X-ray, injections, and excessive manipulations should be avoided. This is not true only for terminal babies, but for all those present in the neonatal intensive care unit, who can receive undue overtreatment and overstimulations [16].

Moreover, strict recommendations are given for the spaces around the incubator of each child. The Committee to Establish Recommended Standards for Newborn ICU Design so says: "Each infant space shall contain a minimum of 120 ft^2 (11.2 m^2) of clear floor space, excluding handwashing stations, columns and aisles. Within this space, there shall be sufficient furnishing to allow a parent to stay seated, reclining or fully recumbent at the bedside" [17]. The presence of parents is fundamental, as well as the skin-to-skin contact, and all the maneuvers apt to reduce pain.

25.4 Parents' Advice

The care of the parents of children and babies is essential in palliative care. Their opinions and advice about their baby's health and concerns are essential. Too often parents are pushed aside, expelled from childcare, at most superficially and quickly informed or left to wait for few and sparse words to get some news. Parents of chronically ill children often experience social isolation, both due to time spent in the hospital, and to a lack of solidariety from the outside world: even their friends marginalizes them, uncertain and scared of talking with them [18]. As a result, parents, and sometimes hospitalized children, often develop close relationships with their peers - parents, and children - in the ICU. Through conversations in the common rooms, or through social media, the parents of the hospitalized children interact with each other [19]: intimacy and almost friendship is created between families united by the period of hospitalization in intensive care. It therefore happens that parents are aware of the developments and progress of other children. A child's loss or setback can profoundly affect another child or their family. Witnessing traumatic events in the other family sharing their own child's room can have various consequences, ranging from post-traumatic stress to the development of comorbidities [20]. It may therefore happen that parents ask the doctor about the procedures on other children. Here is an important point, because neither should one respond unkindly, nor should one violate the privacy of the other family: one should be cautious but never rude, respecting the privacy of other patients, but aware of one family's feelings and concerns for the other.

There is something more: parents should not be overloaded with new stress (bureaucracy, long waits, humiliations) and have the right to be housed next to their child night and day; they should not experience a marked collapse in their role as responsible for their child, due to the difference between what they do at home and what they can do in the hospital [21]. This can lead to a sense of anxiety and frustration [22].

Parents are a support to their children's care, but they are often considered an obstacle or "ghosts", that have no use in that ward. Parents know their children's unique history, unique traits, and the type of usual care their children get; this can be a valuable support to doctors, who get profit from asking the family what they think is best for their children and what is most important to them: children can express anxiety, pain, and joy in ways that only parents who know them intimately can decipher.

25.5 Abundance Medicine

It is common to believe that good health care means good cost/benefit ratio: the maximum patients' satisfaction with the lowest money investment [23]. Several clues show that this should not be an absolute tenet: health care is not only economy; health is the blooming of the person, and it is one of those few areas—along with transport and building safety, police services, and education—where the word "sparing" is somehow inappropriate. You should not generically spare on healthcare, in particular in delicate situations such as end-of-life settings. Here below, we'll see where sparing in intensive care health systems is possible, and where it is utterly wrong.

25.5.1 Healthcare Waste: Defensive Medicine

Today, health care often wastes drugs, personnel, tools, and hospitalizations; the excess of tests, instead of guaranteeing a diagnosis, is often a cause of waste as well:

too many useless tests often give borderline or false-positive results that require other tests and so on, starting a voyage called the "Ulysses syndrome" [24, 25]. Moreover, the response that healthcare systems give to their fail (investments in healthcare soar while public satisfaction plummets) is the multiplication of protocols and procedures; protocols are useful but they are too many, redundant and aimed often only to demonstrate an activity in the department. And this has a cost of time and personnel.

The defensive medicine is the practice of recommending diagnostic tests or medical treatments that are not necessarily the best option for the patient, but an option that mainly protects the physician against the patient as potential plaintiff [26]. Defensive medicine is a reaction to the rising costs of malpractice insurance premiums and patients' biases on suing for missed or delayed diagnosis or treatment, but never for overtreatment. Worldwide physicians are at the highest risk of being sued, and overtreatment is common. Physicians order tests and sometimes avoid treating high-risk patients (when they have a choice to do it) to reduce their exposure to lawsuits; otherwise, they are to discontinue practicing because of high insurance premiums (Fig. 25.1) [27].

Fig. 25.1 Abundance medicine. Unnecessary tests and time-wasting reunions are an obstacle for the availability of the budget. On the converse, personnel's motivation and improvement of the hospitals promote the correct fruition of the budget. Avoiding the SUV effect, we can save money and improve the total clinical performance

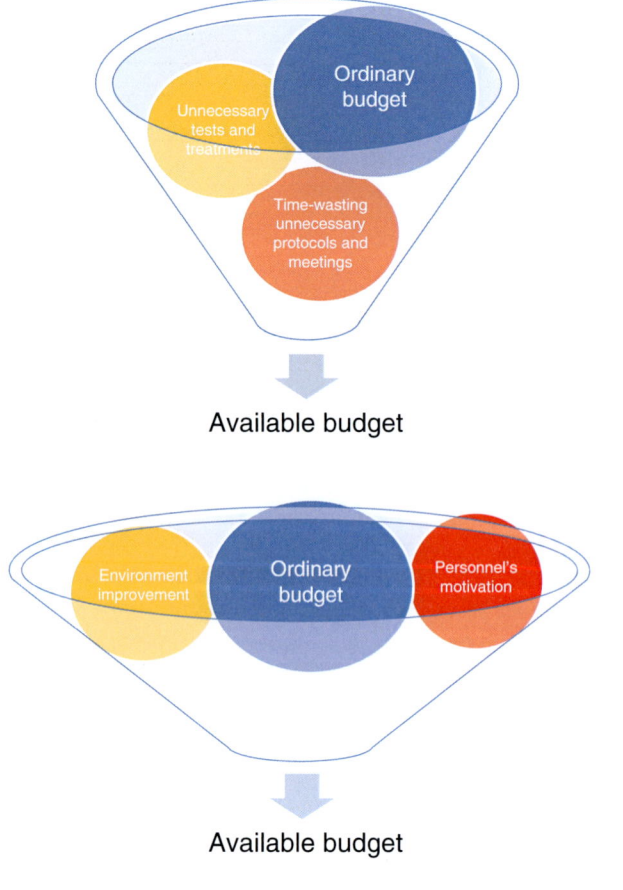

25.5.2 The SUV Effect

The SUV effect [28] is the false sense of safety given by the excessive availability of medical tools, drugs, and tests that makes doctors decrease their attention on the patients; in fact, we are witnessing a decrease of the time doctors devote to talk with their patients, and their skills to investigate and diagnose using their senses, namely touch and sight. The SUV effect takes its name from the sense of safety that SUV (an acronym for Sport Urban Vehicle) owners feel while driving such powerful and shielded cars, where any accident is apparently preventable and avoidable by the technique; unfortunately, this makes human attention decrease and casualties soar [29].

These two phenomena (defensive medicine and the SUV effect) cause money waste that might be avoided. But what can these savings be invested into, to produce a good healthcare?

25.5.3 Abundance Medicine

The new frontier of health care is "tailored" medicine. We call it "abundance medicine", because abundance is what is needed by the patient, namely by the sickest ones. Why should abundance be a prerogative of those who are healthy or only of those who can buy it? It is not a utopia, it is more and more often reported by specialized literature, which speaks of personalized medicine, of holistic cures, that consider not just an apparatus or a disease, but the whole person [30]. We can describe this concept with an example taken from neonatology. A pioneer in the field, the Australian Heidelise Als, has created and disseminated an individualized evaluation system centered on the single newborn and single family, in order to direct the care on the child's sub-system—autonomic, vegetative, behavioral systems—which shows more fragility. This evaluation and treatment system, known with the acronym NIDCAP (Neonatal Individualized Developmental Care Assessment Program), is increasingly followed worldwide: by using it, one understands how to treat babies, respecting their rhythms and needs across their hospitalization; various studies have shown with the use of magnetic resonance that the brain grows more mature and less damaged in children who have received this approach [31]. Sunny Anand, the pioneer in pediatric pain therapy, expresses himself on NIDCAP, while talking about another form of individualized treatment of neonatal pain, the "sensorial saturation": "These approaches provide great attention and commitment to the comfort of the child. Thus, we know how to express empathy for children who receive painful interventions in the hospital" [32].

Heidelise Als was present at the international congress organized by the scientific association "Caring Essentials" held in February 2019 in Brugge (Belgium), aimed at indicating how to overcome the psychological and organic traumas caused by illness and hospitalization to children in neonatal intensive care units, through a personalized treatment, which combines pharmacologic approaches with music therapy, maternal care, and respect of babies' sleep rhythms. The main message of the congress was that personalized cures are fundamental for the little baby, but they also benefit the staff in terms of less stress and burnout prevention. Counterintuitively, they save time and also save the costs of redundant exams or superfluous therapies, by focusing the attention of the staff on the essentials. Treating a child with mother's cuddles—the aforementioned "sensorial saturation"—during a blood drawing not only makes one feel less ill, but also makes the withdrawal faster and easier for the operators [33].

Thus, a myth collapses: that good health care is the one that achieves the utmost results with the least expense. But economy is just one of the parameters to judge healthcare: it should be judged also on the abundance of satisfaction it produces in the patient.

The correct direction for investing in health care and in the intensive care is investing in staff motivation and in the care of the patient's environment, to make everyone feel a little better, more serene, and not just tied to rigid timetables and job profiles.

- Happier personnel are more efficient, more intuitive; and a patient who feels comfortable has often a quicker recover.
- Investing in better hospitals, in personalized timetables for visits, tests, meals, and sleep improves the speed of patients' recovery and soars their satisfaction.

Economy and devoted care of the patient are not two uncommunicable settings: without attention to wastes, healthcare would be shallow, and without a devoted care of the patient it would be an industry.

Personnel motivation is among the goals for a better health care, as promoted by the WHO [34] and should be the center of any intensive care, as well as a better environment for patients, families, and caregivers.

We call "abundance medicine" the medical system that knows the wastes to be cut, and simultaneously acknowledges the importance of implementing and funding those sectors that give motivation and hope to both caregivers and patients. The abundance medicine enhances the human factor: the possibilities of the sick, and the healing powers of a comfortable environment; it also avoids wastes as well as the upsetting and cold medical bureaucracy. Abundance is not "excess" or "waste," as it may seem at a shallow sight; its real sense is "exuberance," a word that derives from the latin "ex" ("from") and "ubera" ("breasts"), meaning "having in the breast so much milk to give." The "abundance healthcare" is to be exuberant in time it devotes to the patient, beyond what is written in the contracts; and exuberant in its humanity. A nurse or a physician devoted to their patients and not only to their job list, would guarantee a thorough use of the available resources, sparing money and time. It is this abundance of humanity that must be enhanced, in a world of corporate medicine where we are invited to limit ourselves to respond to schedules and contractual rules rather than to our patients.

References

1. Kaye EC, Rubenstein J, Levine D, Baker JN, Dabbs D, Friebert SE. Pediatric palliative care in the community. CA Cancer J Clin. 2015;65(4):316–33.
2. Pritchard M, Burghen E, Srivastava DK, et al. Cancer-related symptoms most concerning to parents during the last week and last day of their child's life. Pediatrics. 2008;121:e1301–9.

References

3. Quill TE, Abernethy AP. Generalist plus specialist palliative care—creating a more sustainable model. N Engl J Med. 2013;368:1173–5.
4. Short SR, Thienprayoon R. Pediatric palliative care in the intensive care unit and questions of quality: a review of the determinants and mechanisms of high-quality palliative care in the pediatric intensive care unit (PICU). Transl Pediatr. 2018;7(4):326–43. https://doi.org/10.21037/tp.2018.09.11.
5. Greenfield DK, Carter B, Harrop DE, Jassal DS, Bayliss MJ, Renton DK, Holley DS, Howard DRF, Johnson MM, Liossi C. Healthcare professionals' experiences of the barriers and facilitators to paediatric pain management in the community at end-of-life: a qualitative interview study. J Pain Symptom Manage. 2022;63(1):98–105. https://doi.org/10.1016/j.jpainsymman.2021.06.026.
6. Cardoso SB, Oliveira ICDS, Souza TV, SAD C. Pediatric intensive care unit: reflection in the light of Florence Nightingale's Environmental Theory. Rev Bras Enferm. 2021;74(5):e20201267. https://doi.org/10.1590/0034-7167-2020-1267.
7. Nightingale F. Notas sobre enfermagem: o que é e o que não é. São Paulo: Cortez; 1989.
8. Terzi B, Azizoğlu F, Polat Ş, Kaya N, İşsever H. The effects of noise levels on nurses in intensive care units. Nurs Crit Care. 2019;24(5):299–305. https://doi.org/10.1111/nicc.12414. Epub 2019 Feb 28.
9. The Pediatric Intensive Care Society. Appendices to the standards for the care of critically ill children. 2010. Accessed on May 5th 2022. https://pccsociety.uk/wp-content/uploads/2015/10/PICS_Standards_Appendix_2010.pdf.
10. Santos PM, Silva JOM, Makuch DMV, Souza AB, Silva LF, Depiant JRB. A percepção da criança hospitalizada quanto ao ambiente da unidade de terapia intensiva pediátrica. Rev Inic Cient Ext [Internet]. 2020 [cited 2020 Sep 7];3(1):331-340. Available from: https://revistasfacesa.senaaires.com.br/index.php/iniciacao-cientifica/article/view/19
11. HBN. 04-02 Critical care units. 2013. https://www.thenbs.com/PublicationIndex/documents/details?Pub=NHS&DocID=303350
12. Stroustrup A, Bragg JB, Spear EA, Aguiar A, Zimmerman E, Isler JR, Busgang SA, Curtin PC, Gennings C, Andra SS, Arora M. Cohort profile: the neonatal intensive care unit hospital exposures and long-term health (NICU-HEALTH) cohort, a prospective preterm birth cohort in new York City. BMJ Open. 2019;9(11):e032758. https://doi.org/10.1136/bmjopen-2019-032758.
13. Bickle-Graz M, Tolsa JF, Fischer Fumeaux CJ. Phthalates in the NICU: a survey. Arch Dis Child Fetal Neonatal Ed. 2020;105(1):110–1. https://doi.org/10.1136/archdischild-2019-317582. Epub 2019 Sep 10.
14. Verderber S, Gray S, Suresh-Kumar S, Kercz D, Parshuram C. Intensive care unit built environments: a comprehensive literature review (2005-2020). HERD. 2021;14(4):368–415. https://doi.org/10.1177/19375867211009273.
15. Bellieni CV, Buonocore G, Pinto I, Stacchini N, Cordelli DM, Bagnoli F. Use of sound-absorbing panel to reduce noisy incubator reverberating effects. Biol Neonate. 2003;84(4):293–6. https://doi.org/10.1159/000073637.
16. Baumann T. Unnecessary health care. 2021. https://www.paediatrieschweiz.ch/?lang=de
17. White RD. Recommended NICU design standards and the physical environment of the NICU. J Perinatol. 2013;33 Suppl 1:S1.
18. Hickerton CL, Aitken M, Hodgson J, Delatycki MB. "Did you find that out in time?": new life trajectories of parents who choose to continue a pregnancy where a genetic disorder is diagnosed or likely. Am J Med Genet A. 2012;158A(2):373–83.
19. Khouri JS, McCheyne MJ, Morrison CS. #Cleft: the use of social media amongst parents of infants with clefts. Cleft Palate Craniofac J. 2018;55(7):974–6. https://doi.org/10.1597/16-156. Epub 2018 Feb 22.
20. Handley TE, Kelly BJ, Lewin TJ, et al. Long-term effects of lifetime trauma exposure in a rural community sample. BMC Public Health. 2015;15:1176.
21. Graham RJ, Pemstein DM, Curley MA. Experiencing the pediatric intensive care unit: perspective from parents of children with severe antecedent disabilities. Crit Care Med. 2009;37(6):2064–70. https://doi.org/10.1097/CCM.0b013e3181a00578.

22. Baird J, Rehm RS, Hinds PS, Baggott C, Davies B. Do you know my child? Continuity of nursing care in the pediatric intensive care unit. Nurs Res. 2016;65(2):142–50. https://doi.org/10.1097/NNR.0000000000000135.
23. Birth S, Donaldson C. Applications of cost-benefit analysis to health care: departures from welfare economic theory. J Health Econ. 1987;6(3):211–25.
24. Parmar MS. Ulysses syndrome and the COVID-19 pandemic. South Med J. 2021;114(5):317–8.
25. Rang M. The Ulysses syndrome. Can Med Assoc J. 1972;106(2):122–3.
26. Kattel P. Defensive medicine: is it legitimate or immoral? J Nepal Health Res Counc. 2019;16(41):483–5.
27. Studdert DM, Mello MM, Sage WM, DesRoches CM, Peugh J, Zapert K, Brennan TA. Defensive medicine among high-risk specialist physicians in a volatile malpractice environment. JAMA. 2005;293(21):2609–17.
28. Bellieni CV, Buonocore G. What we do in neonatal analgesia overshadows how we do it. Acta Paediatr. 2018;107(3):388–90.
29. Wallner P, Wanka A, Hutter HP. SUV driving "masculinizes" risk behavior in females: a public health challenge. Wien Klin Wochenschr. 2017;129(17–18):625–9.
30. Jasemi M, Valizadeh L, Zamanzadeh V, Keogh B. A concept analysis of holistic care by hybrid model. Indian J Palliat Care. 2017;23(1):71–80.
31. Als H, Duffy FH, McAnulty G, Butler SC, Lightbody L, Kosta S, Weisenfeld NI, Robertson R, Parad RB, Ringer SA, Blickman JG, Zurakowski D, Warfield SK. NIDCAP improves brain function and structure in preterm infants with severe intrauterine growth restriction. J Perinatol. 2012;32(10):797–803.
32. Anand KJ, Hall RW. Love, pain, and intensive care. Pediatrics. 2008;121(4):825–7.
33. Locatelli C, Bellieni CV. Sensorial saturation and neonatal pain: a review. J Matern Fetal Neonatal Med. 2018;31(23):3209–13.
34. World Health Organization, Organisation for Economic Co-operation and Development, and The World Bank: delivering quality health services: a global imperative for universal health coverage. Geneva; 2018. http://apps.who.int/iris/bitstream/handle/10665/272465/9789241513906-eng.pdf

Conclusion

The time we are living in is the time of the stage: one is integrated into the society only if one knows how to stay on the scene. It is the time that Marcuse called the time of the monads, but which Heidegger resized by calling it the time of chatter.

The life of the terminal child, the life of palliative care is a world out of this world of jostling to prevail and to excel, but it is a world more real than the other which has lost sight of reality and lives only in the performance-related anxiety, so much so that it is infested of adolescent depression and severe children's hyperactivity.

In the frantic world longing for supremacy, attention deficit prevails; in the world of palliative care, there is a surplus of attention. So, it is here that paradoxically the human factor is recovered, even in the harshness of the end-of-life and of the disease. There we recover the sense of care and the sense of curiosity, both idioms that come from the Latin word "cor" which means heart.

I wish all those who fight their battle of illness and end of life, be they doctors, nurses, children, or parents, to recover from this difficult situation and learn to get closer to their heart.

Printed by Books on Demand, Germany